The Pediatric Foot and Ankle

Guest Editor

RAYMOND J. SULLIVAN, MD

FOOT AND ANKLE CLINICS

Consulting Editor
MARK S. MYERSON, MD

June 2010 • Volume 15 • Number 2

SAUNDERS an imprint of ELSEVIER, Inc.

W.B. SAUNDERS COMPANY
A Division of Elsevier Inc.

1600 John F. Kennedy Blvd. • Suite 1800 • Philadelphia, PA 19103-2899

http://www.theclinics.com

FOOT AND ANKLE CLINICS Volume 15, Number 2
June 2010 ISSN 1083-7515, ISBN-13: 978-1-4377-1821-8

Editor: Debora Dellapena
Developmental Editor: Donald Mumford

Foot and Ankle Clinics (ISSN 1083-7515) is published quarterly by Elsevier, Inc., 360 Park Avenue South, New York, NY 10010-1710. Months of issue are March, June, September, and December. Periodicals postage paid at New York, NY, and additional mailing offices. Subscription price per year is $253.00 (US individuals), $340.00 (US institutions), $128.00 (US students), $283.00 (Canadian individuals), $402.00 (Canadian institutions), $175.00 (Canadian students), $364.00 (foreign individuals), $402.00 (foreign institutions), and $175.00 (foreign students). To receive student/resident rate, orders must be accompanied by name of affiliated institution, date of term, and the *signature* of program/residency coordinator on institution letterhead. Orders will be billed at individual rate until proof of status is received. Foreign air speed delivery is included in all *Clinics* subscription prices. All prices are subject to change without notice. **POSTMASTER:** Send address changes to *Foot and Ankle Clinics*, Elsevier Health Sciences Division, Subscription Customer Service, 3251 Riverport Lane, Maryland Heights, MO 63043. **Customer Service: 1-800-654-2452 (US and Canada). From outside of the United States and Canada, call 314-447-8871. Fax: 314-417-8029. E-mail: JournalsCustomerService-usa@ elsevier.com (for print support); JournalsOnlineSupport-usa@elsevier.com (for online support).**

Reprints. For copies of 100 or more, of articles in this publication, please contact the Commercial Reprints Department, Elsevier Inc., 360 Park Avenue South, New York, NY 10010-1710. Tel.: 212-633-3812; Fax: 212-462-1935; E-mail: reprints@elsevier.com.

Printed and bound by CPI Group (UK) Ltd, Croydon, CR0 4YY

Transferred to Digital Print 2011

Contributors

CONSULTING EDITOR

MARK S. MYERSON, MD
Director, The Institute for Foot and Ankle Reconstruction at Mercy, Mercy Medical Center, Baltimore, Maryland

GUEST EDITOR

RAYMOND J. SULLIVAN, MD
Clinical Associate Professor, Department of Orthopedics, University of Connecticut; Orthopedic Associates of Hartford, Farmington, Connecticut

AUTHORS

FERNÁNDO ÁLVAREZ, MD
Head of Foot and Ankle Unit, Department of Orthopedic Surgery, Hospital San Rafael, Barcelona, Spain

JAMES W. BRODSKY, MD
Director, Foot and Ankle Surgery Fellowship Program, Baylor University Medical Center; Clinical Professor of Orthopaedic Surgery, University of Texas Southwestern Medical School, Dallas, Texas

JAMES D.F. CALDER, MD, FRCS (Tr&Orth), FFSEM(UK)
Consultant Orthopaedic Surgeon, Department of Trauma and Orthopaedic Surgery, Basingstoke and North Hampshire Hospitals NHS Foundation Trust, Imperial College School of Medicine Science and Technology, Charing Cross Hospital, London, United Kingdom

RICHARD S. DAVIDSON, MD
Associate Professor Pediatric Orthopedics, Department of Orthopaedic Surgery, The University of Pennsylvania, School of Medicine, The Children's Hospital of Philadelphia; Shriners Hospital, Philadelphia, Pennsylvania

PABLO FERNÁNDEZ DE RETANA, MD
Head of Orthopedic Surgery, Department of Orthopedic Surgery, Hospital San Rafael, Barcelona, Spain

SUNIL DHAR, MBBS, MS, MCh Orth, FRCS, FRCS Ed Orth
Consultant Trauma and Orthopaedic Surgeon, Department of Trauma and Orthopaedics, Nottingham University Hospitals, Queen's Medical Centre Campus, Nottingham, United Kingdom

PAUL T. FORTIN, MD
Attending, Department of Orthopaedics, William Beaumont Hospital; Orthopaedic Foot and Ankle Surgery, Oakland Orthopaedic Surgeons, Royal Oak, Michigan

B. DAVID HORN, MD
Assistant Professor of Clinical Orthopaedic Surgery, Department of Orthopaedic Surgery, The University of Pennsylvania School of Medicine, The Children's Hospital of Philadelphia, Philadelphia, Pennsylvania

JULIE KOHLS-GATZOULIS, FRCS (Tr&Orth)
Department of Trauma and Orthopaedic Surgery, Royal Surrey County Hospital, Guildford, United Kingdom

HARISH V. KURUP, MS(Orth), FRCS (Orth)
Paediatric Orthopaedic Fellow, Department of Paediatric Orthopaedics, Southampton University Hospital, Southampton, Hampshire, United Kingdom

JOHN Y. KWON, MD
Department of Orthopaedic Surgery; Clinical Instructor, Harvard Medical School, Massachusetts General Hospital, Boston, Massachusetts

ZACHARY C. LEONARD, MD
Resident, Department of Orthopaedics, William Beaumont Hospital, Royal Oak, Michigan

MARK S. MYERSON, MD
Director, The Institute for Foot and Ankle Reconstruction at Mercy, Mercy Medical Center, Baltimore, Maryland

MATTHEW C. SOLAN, FRCS (Tr&Orth)
Department of Trauma and Orthopaedic Surgery, Royal Surrey County Hospital, Guildford, United Kingdom

JULIE STEBBINS, DPhil, SRCS, CSci, MIPEM
Clinical Scientist, Oxford Gait Laboratory, Nuffield Orthopaedic Centre, Headington, Oxford, United Kingdom

MICHAEL M. STEPHENS, MSc (Bioeng), FRCSI
Professor, Department of Orthopaedic Surgery, Children's University Hospital, Dublin, Ireland

TIM THEOLOGIS, MD, MSc, PhD, FRCS
Consultant Orthopaedic Surgeon, Nuffield Orthopaedic Centre, Headington, Oxford, United Kingdom

MICHAEL G. UGLOW, FRCS (Tr&Orth)
Consultant Orthopaedic Surgeon, Department of Paediatric Orthopaedics, Southampton University Hospital, Southampton, Hampshire, United Kingdom

RAMÓN VILADOT, MD
Clínica Tres Torres, Barcelona, Spain

HTWE ZAW, FRCS (Tr&Orth)
Fellow in Orthopaedic Surgery, Department of Trauma and Orthopaedic Surgery, Basingstoke and North Hampshire Hospitals NHS Foundation Trust, Basingstoke, United Kingdom

Contents

Preface   ix

Raymond J. Sullivan

Current Treatment of Clubfoot in Infancy and Childhood   235

B. David Horn and Richard S. Davidson

Clubfoot is one of the most common congenital anomalies seen in newborns and children. Although the cause is unknown, strides have recently been made in uncovering the etiology causes of clubfoot. In the last decade, the treatment of clubfoot has undergone a significant change with a shift away from extensive operative intervention to a less invasive approach. Long-term residual deformity and pain from surgically corrected club feet still continues to occur and presents diagnostic and therapeutic challenges for the orthopedic surgeon.

Residual Clubfoot in Children   245

Michael G. Uglow and Harish V. Kurup

The deformities encountered in any patient who has residual clubfoot comprise various degrees of equinus, varus, adduction, supination, cavus, and toe deformity. Joint flexibility or stiffness, tarsal dysmorphism, articular incongruence, and progressive degrees of degeneration may be present. Add to this the scars of previous attempts at correction and various etiologic factors, and surgeons can find that treatment solutions are far from straightforward. A philosophy of careful history, examination, investigation, and surgery à la carte will provide a safe foundation for treating patients who have these often complex and difficult problems. A surgical strategy progressing from proximal to distal, performing soft tissue surgery before fixed deformity occurs, extra-articular osteotomies to correct bony deformity, and augmentation with rebalancing of soft tissue–deforming forces will help improve pain and function for many patients. Joint fusions should be reserved as a last salvage option to avoid future degeneration of adjacent joints.

Ilizarov External Fixation in the Correction of Severe Pediatric Foot and Ankle Deformities   265

Sunil Dhar

Most of the evidence to date on the Ilizarov method in the management of complex foot and ankle deformities in children is based on expert opinion and retrospective case series. Often the technique is used as a salvage option where conventional techniques are inappropriate or have failed. The decision to use the Ilizarov external fixator to an alternative technique depends on several issues: complexity of the pathology, patient compliance, surgeon skills, and the capacity of the institution to manage patients with multidisciplinary requirements. Nevertheless, the Ilizarov method has proved to be a valuable tool for the satisfactory management of many previously unresolved clinical problems. With greater experience and further developments, the exact place of this powerful treatment modality will become clearer and even more successful.

The Adult Sequelae of Treated Congenital Clubfoot   287

James W. Brodsky

There are limited studies about the incidence, nature, and severity of symptoms in adults with treated clubfoot; the rate at which symptoms increase and function diminishes with advancing age; and the appropriate treatments. One of the principles of treatment of these patients includes recognition that no one description of deformities applies to all cases of painful deformity in adults after childhood treatment of congenital clubfoot. There is a spectrum of the types of deformity and a range of severity among these that must be taken into account in the decision making regarding treatment. Although the level of symptoms is very variable and ankle and hindfoot arthrodeses have the disadvantage of increasing mechanical stress and subsequent arthritis in the midfoot, arthrodesis and, to a lesser degree, osteotomy remain the mainstays of surgical reconstruction in the adult with painful deformity after treatment of congenital talipes equinovarus.

Idiopathic Toe Walking and Contractures of the Triceps Surae   297

Matthew C. Solan, Julie Kohls-Gatzoulis, and Michael M. Stephens

Toe walking is a common feature in immature gait and is considered normal up to 3 years of age. As walking ability improves, initial contact is made with the heel. Toe-walkers will stand out as different once heel-strike is achieved by most of their peers. This difference gives rise to parental concern. Therefore toe-walkers are often referred at 3 years of age. This article examines the evidence for the management of children who have idiopathic toe walking and reviews the literature on surgery for the lengthening of a calf contracture.

Management of the Flexible Flat Foot in the Child: A Focus on the Use
of Osteotomies for Correction   309

John Y. Kwon and Mark S. Myerson

Pes planus, commonly referred as flat foot, is a combination of foot and ankle deformities. When faced with this deformity in children, the treating surgeon should use a systematic method for evaluation to distinguish normal variation from true pathology, as well as conditions that have a benign natural history versus those that may lead to significant disability if left untreated. Certain deformities will inevitably worsen and therefore require surgery. Common sense clearly supports the indication for a simple procedure, such as an arthroereisis or an osteotomy, performed in the young child as opposed to an arthrodesis in older adolescence or adulthood as the foot becomes more rigid. Such approaches and other issues are discussed in this article.

Subtalar Arthroereisis in Pediatric Flatfoot Reconstruction   323

Pablo Fernández de Retana, Fernándo Álvarez, and Ramón Viladot

Pediatric and juvenile flatfoot is a common problem in childhood, present in one in nine children. The morphologic characteristics of this condition are heel valgus and flattening of the medial longitudinal arch. Other characteristics are usually observed, such as supination and abduction of the forefoot, tightening of the Achilles tendon, and hypertonia of the peroneal muscles. Most children with flatfoot will undergo spontaneous correction or become asymptomatic; those that are symptomatic require treatment. Subtalar arthroereisis, often combined with Achilles tendon lengthening, is a simple and effective way to treat flexible flatfoot in children. Mid- and long-term results are good, and the procedure does not prevent future treatments.

Adolescent Accessory Navicular   337

Zachary C. Leonard and Paul T. Fortin

Accessory tarsal navicular is a common anomaly in the human foot. It should be in the differential of medial foot pain. A proper history and physical, along with imaging modalities, can lead to the diagnosis. Often, classification of the ossicle and amount of morbidity guide treatment. Nonsurgical measures can provide relief. A variety of surgical procedures have been used with good results. Our preferred method is excision for small ossicles and segmental fusion after removal of the synchondrosis for large ossicles. In addition, pes planovalgus deformities need to be addressed concomitantly.

Tarsal Coalitions   349

Htwe Zaw and James D.F. Calder

A tarsal coalition is an aberrant union between two or more tarsal bones and can be classified as osseous (synostosis) or nonosseous (cartilaginous [synchondrosis] or fibrous [syndesmosis]). This union may be complete or partial and the joints in the hindfoot and midfoot are most commonly affected. The resulting abnormal articulation presents as a noncorrectable flat foot, usually during adolescence, leading to accelerated degeneration within adjacent joints. An understanding of the condition and presenting symptoms enable the clinician to correctly diagnose and initiate appropriate treatment. This review discusses the evidence-based literature on the cause, diagnosis, and current management of tarsal coalition.

The Use of Gait Analysis in the Treatment of Pediatric Foot and Ankle Disorders   365

Tim Theologis and Julie Stebbins

Assessment of foot pathology during walking should form an integral part of the clinical evaluation of children. Simple observation and video recording have limitations and are not quantifiable. Three-dimensional analysis of foot motion during walking can provide invaluable information on the dynamic function of the foot and can contribute to clinical decision making. As motion analysis technology advances, the accuracy and reliability of the dynamic assessment of the foot during walking will increase further, allowing clinicians to rely confidently on this information during patient assessment and the study of treatment outcomes. It is logical to expect that objective and quantifiable assessment of gait should be undertaken before and after treatment that sets gait improvement as one of its aims.

Index   383

FORTHCOMING ISSUES

September 2010
Infection, Ischemia and Amputation
Michael S. Pinzur, MD, *Guest Editor*

December 2010
Orthobiologic Concepts in Foot and Ankle
Stuart D. Miller, MD, *Guest Editor*

RECENT ISSUES

March 2010
Traumatic Foot and Ankle Injuries Related
to Recent International Conflicts
Eric M. Bluman, MD, PhD,
and James R. Ficke, MD, *Guest Editors*

December 2009
Achilles Tendon
G. Andrew Murphy, MD, *Guest Editor*

September 2009
Correction of Multiplanar Deformity
of the Foot and Ankle
Anish R. Kadakia, MD, *Guest Editor*

THE CLINICS ARE NOW AVAILABLE ONLINE!

Access your subscription at:
www.theclinics.com

Preface

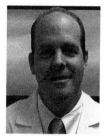

Raymond J. Sullivan, MD
Guest Editor

A wise man once said, *"The child's foot is not just a smaller version of the adult foot."*[1]

This issue of *Foot and Ankle Clinics of North America* has an update of the excellent work published in a previous edition of *Foot and Ankle Clinics of North America* in 1998 with Dr Richard Davidson as the guest editor. The objective of the present issue was to update the techniques of clubfoot, tarsal coalition, and pediatric flat foot reconstruction, as well as to indicate how the changes in surgical techniques have affected long-term outcomes and the differences in adult reconstructions secondarily. An article on gait analysis and how these techniques can be used in surgical planning is included.

I would like to thank the international authors for their contributions. I am especially grateful to Drs Mark Myerson and Richard Davidson, my fellowship directors and mentors, for their contributions to this edition.

Raymond J. Sullivan, MD
Department of Orthopedics, University of Connecticut
Orthopedic Associates of Hartford
499 Farmington Avenue, Farmington
CT 06032, USA

E-mail address:
pedsfoot@aol.com

---

[1] Richardson RS, Foreword. Foot and Ankle Clinics 1998;3:13.

Foot Ankle Clin N Am 15 (2010) ix
doi:10.1016/j.fcl.2010.04.005

Current Treatment of Clubfoot in Infancy and Childhood

B. David Horn, MD[a],*, Richard S. Davidson, MD[a,b]

KEYWORDS

• Clubfoot • Ponseti technique • Serial casting • Tenotomy

The incidence of clubfoot is 1 in 1000 live births and exhibits considerable variation among different ethnic populations.[1,2] Ethnic Chinese have a very low incidence of 0.39 per 1000 live births, whereas Hawaiians and Maoris have a very high incidence of approximately 7 per 1000 live births.[3] This variance obviously suggests a genetic influence in the cause of clubfoot.

Clubfoot consists of 4 components, which can be remembered through the acronym CAVE: cavus, forefoot adductus, hindfoot varus, and hindfoot equinus. CAVE also represents the order of correction of a clubfoot when the Ponseti method is used (see later section). The severity at presentation may vary from a mild, flexible clubfoot to a severe, rigid foot. Clubfoot may be associated with known syndromes such as arthrogryposis or myelodysplasia or with other congenital or chromosomal anomalies.[1] Most club feet, however, are classified as idiopathic and occur in isolation. The natural history of untreated clubfoot leads to the lateral aspect and dorsum of the foot becoming weight-bearing surfaces. Hypertrophic calluses develop, and the foot becomes painful with weight bearing. With an untreated clubfoot, regular shoe wear becomes impossible and individuals experience significant disability.

ETIOLOGY

Clubfoot is believed to result from a neuromuscular disorder affecting the foot and ankle. This disorder may be obvious, as in cases of clubfoot associated with myelomeningocele and arthrogryposis, or the clubfoot may be secondary to an as yet unrecognized neuromuscular process, as is suspected in idiopathic clubfoot. The cause of idiopathic clubfoot has been variously ascribed to intrauterine positioning,[4] environmental factors such as secondhand smoke,[5] abnormal muscle and soft tissue, abnormal bone formation, and vascular malformations.[6–8] Despite a study linking

[a] Department of Orthopaedic Surgery, 2nd Floor Wood Center, The University of Pennsylvania School of Medicine, The Children's Hospital of Philadelphia, Philadelphia, PA 19104, USA
[b] Shriners Hospital, Philadelphia, PA 19104, USA
* Corresponding author.
E-mail address: HORND@email.chop.edu

Foot Ankle Clin N Am 15 (2010) 235–243
doi:10.1016/j.fcl.2010.03.003
1083-7515/10/$ – see front matter © 2010 Elsevier Inc. All rights reserved.

clubfoot to early amniocentesis, there is no convincing evidence supporting intra-uterine compression as a cause of clubfoot. Various environmental factors, such as maternal smoking or elevated maternal homocysteine levels, have also been associated with clubfoot.[9,10]

Recent studies have investigated genetic influences in club feet. The genetic cause of club feet has been bolstered by twin concordance studies demonstrating a 33% concordance of club feet in identical twins, but only 3% in fraternal twins and siblings.[11] The exact mode of inheritance of clubfoot is unknown, however. Studies have suggested that club feet may be a result of a single incompletely dominant gene with incomplete penetrance, which may also require the interaction of yet unknown physiologic and environmental factors.[1,12] There is an ongoing search for specific genes that are related to the development of club feet, but to date, no single gene has been identified as a causative factor in idiopathic club feet.

TREATMENT

In the past 10 years, clubfoot treatment has undergone a significant shift away from aggressive surgical correction and toward manipulation accompanied by selective, minimal surgical intervention.[13–15] In the later part of the nineteenth century, clubfoot was corrected by forceful manipulation, using crude devices such as the Thomas wrench. In the midtwentieth century, Kite[16] developed a casting technique involving serial manipulation and casting of the clubfoot. Kite's technique involved sequential correction of all components of the clubfoot. This included abduction of the foot through the midtarsal joints, using the calcaneocuboid joint as a pivot point. Use of the calcaneocuboid joint as a pivot, however, prevented external rotation through the subtalar joint, impeding full correction of the clubfoot's adduction and varus. Kite's technique, therefore, frequently required lengthy periods of casting with treatment times lasting up to 2 years and incomplete correction.[17]

In 1971, Turco[18] published his technique for a 1-stage posterior-medial release of clubfoot accompanied by internal fixation. Comprehensive soft tissue releases rapidly became popular for the treatment of clubfoot. These techniques, although varying in detail, all emphasized a posterior release of the ankle joint and subtalar joint, lengthening of the posterior and medial tendons, and a medial release of the talonavicular joint and subtalar joint.[18,19] Posterolateral ankle and subtalar releases as well as a lateral calcaneocuboid release later were added to the surgical procedure by other investigators.[20,21] These surgeries provided thorough and comprehensive correction of the clubfoot deformity but resulted in many complications, such as neurovascular injury, iatrogenic injury to bone, avascular necrosis of the navicular, wound healing problems, overcorrection, and undercorrection.[22] Long-term studies have also demonstrated the following problems with these extensive surgeries: ankle and subtalar joint stiffness, muscle weakness, arthritis, pain, and residual deformity, with deterioration of the results over time.[23,24]

In the 1940s and 1950s, Ignacio Ponseti began investigating the pathoanatomy of club feet and developed a manipulative method of clubfoot correction that now bears his name. In the last 10 years, the Ponseti technique of clubfoot correction has become the worldwide gold standard for clubfoot correction and obviates extensive surgical release in more than 97% of patients.[14,25,26] This technique relies on a specific sequence of foot manipulation and casting, well-timed minimally invasive surgical intervention, and long-term bracing (with concomitant family involvement and support).[27] The results at intermediate to long-term follow-up seem to support the contention that the Ponseti technique preserves the mobility and correction of the clubfoot while avoiding the complications associated with extensive surgical releases. A retrospective review published in 1995 evaluating 45 patients with 71 club feet at an average age of 34 years demonstrated 78% good to excellent results, with the Ponseti technique.[12]

The general outline of the Ponseti technique includes serial casting ideally started within the first month of life. About 6 to 8 long leg casts are changed every 5 to 7 days to correct the foot's cavus, adductus, and varus. In most patients, this procedure is followed by a percutaneous heel cord tenotomy to correct the equinus contracture. The foot is then recasted for about 3 weeks and then placed in an abduction brace for 3 months full-time, followed by nighttime brace wear until the age of about 4 years. Parental education and cooperation are vital in achieving success with this method.

Casts for the Ponseti technique are applied in accordance with a specific technique.[1,17,25] Long leg casts are used, and although Ponseti describes the use of plaster casts, the use of semirigid fiberglass casting material has been described.[28,29] Ideally, casting should begin within the first few weeks of life. This is to take advantage of the relative elasticity of the soft tissues in the newborn. Casting in most healthy babies begins after discharge from the neonatal nursery, typically within the first 4 weeks of life. Late presentation, however, should not deter from the use of the Ponseti technique because this method has been successfully used in children up to 6 years of age.[30]

The first cast is placed with dorsally directed pressure beneath the first metatarsal to elevate the first ray and correct the cavus, which is invariably present with a clubfoot. The remaining casts take advantage of the anatomy and pathoanatomy of the clubfoot: the clubfoot can be viewed as a rotary subluxation of the midfoot beneath the talus. The talus is held firmly within the mortise by the shape of the ankle joint and its associated ligaments. The calcaneus is firmly bound to the cuboid, navicular, and the rest of the foot by stout ligamentous structures so that the calcaneus and midfoot move as a unit. In the clubfoot, the calcaneus and foot are rotated medially beneath the talus, resulting in foot adduction, supination, and inversion. Correction of the clubfoot, therefore, involves lateral rotation of the calcaneus from its adducted position beneath the talus. This is accomplished by abducting with the forefoot in supination (to lock the joints of the midfoot), using the lateral talar head as a pivot point. Each cast is preceded by stretching and casting the foot into external rotation while gently supinating the foot. This creates gradual external rotation of the foot so that by about the fourth cast, the thigh foot angle should be about 50° as the calcaneus abducts from beneath the talus (**Fig. 1**).

At this point, a decision should be made regarding the correction of the ankle equinus. Most patients would require surgical treatment for the equinus contracture.[13,14] If 10° to 15° of ankle dorsiflexion with the knee extended and the heel in varus can be achieved through manipulation and casting alone, then the patient may be ready for a foot abduction orthosis without a heel cord tenotomy. When an Achilles tenotomy is required, the procedure may be performed in younger infants in the outpatient clinic under local anesthesia or in the operating room under general anesthesia.[17,31,32] The use of a general anesthetic may also allow for a release of the posterior ankle and subtalar joint if contractures of those structures are impeding ankle dorsiflexion. The ankle tenotomy is typically performed about 1 to 1.5 cm proximal to the insertion of the Achilles tendon on the calcaneus. A small blade is percutaneously inserted from the medial aspect of the tendon, and a complete tenotomy performed. A "pop" should be heard or felt, and a successful tenotomy is confirmed by ankle dorsiflexion 10° to 15° with the knee in extension and the heel in varus. After the procedure, a final clubfoot cast is placed with the foot abducted 70° and dorsiflexed 5° to 10°. This

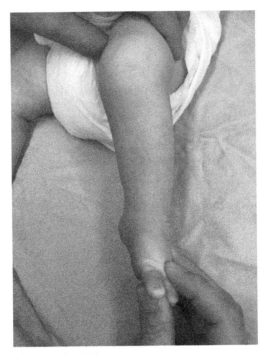

Fig. 1. Supination and external rotation.

last cast is maintained for 3 weeks. After 3 weeks in the final cast the child is placed in a foot abduction orthosis. The clubfoot side is externally rotated 70°, whereas the normal foot (if a unilateral clubfoot) is externally rotated about 30° to 40°. The foot abduction orthosis is worn full-time (23 hours daily) for 3 months and then at nighttime and nap time until the patient is 4 years of age.

Parental and family education is an integral component of the Ponseti clubfoot treatment method, particularly when it comes to brace wear. The brace is vital in maintaining correction of the foot. Several studies have demonstrated that success of the Ponseti technique is directly related to brace compliance and tolerance.[14,23,33,34] Increasing difficulty with brace wear is often an early sign of relapse and may be related to worsening hindfoot varus and equinus.

Relapse or residual deformity occurs in up to 35% of patients.[14,35] Early relapses can often successfully be treated with repeat serial casting. If, after repeat casting, ankle dorsiflexion is still less than about 15°, consideration should be given to performing repeat heel cord tenotomy. Relapses in children older than about 18 months typically require more extensive soft tissue releases. A medial cuneiform opening wedge osteotomy with or without a closing wedge cuboid osteotomy may be useful in children older than 3 to 4 years with a relapse or recurrence of their club feet.

About 30% of children treated with the Ponseti technique demonstrate, by about 3 to 4 years of age, recurrent hindfoot varus coupled with dynamic forefoot supination while walking. This condition may be successfully treated with repeat serial casting to correct the heel varus and foot adduction, followed by a transfer of the tibialis anterior tendon.[35] This procedure is a complete transfer of the tibialis anterior tendon to the lateral-most cuneiform and can be done without making an incision in the anterior leg and tracing the tendon up to its origin. The tendon should remain beneath the extensor retinaculum (to prevent bowstringing) and may be attached to the bone either with an absorbable pull-through suture tied over a button or with a suture anchor. If residual ankle equinus is present, the transfer can be combined with a repeat heel cord lengthening or gastrocsoleus recession. Postoperatively, the foot is placed in a cast for 6 weeks, followed by an ankle foot orthosis for 3 to 6 months. Physical therapy for stretching, range of motion, and strengthening and instruction in a home exercise program may also be useful after this procedure.

Although the Ponseti technique was originally described for idiopathic club feet, its use has been extended to club feet associated with neuromuscular diseases such as myelomeningocele and arthrogryposis. Serial casting with this technique in children with these conditions has been shown, at least in short-term follow-up, to result in satisfactory correction, decreasing the need for extensive surgical releases.[36–38] In addition, there is a subset of patients with idiopathic club feet whose feet are short, are fatter than expected, have a short first ray, and have a deep transverse plantar crease. These patients are considered to have an atypical clubfoot.[15] The Ponseti technique may be used successfully in these patients; however, the technique needs to be modified by increasing the duration of casting and changing the force and direction of manipulation.[15]

A second, minimally invasive method of clubfoot treatment that has also become popular in the last 10 years is known as the functional method. This technique, developed by Masse and Bensahel and known colloquially as the French method, relies on daily manipulations and stretching of a newborn's clubfoot by a trained physical therapist.[17,39] This treatment is based on the idea that the primary pathoanatomy in clubfoot is a tight fibrosis medially in the midfoot and posterior tibialis muscle as well as peroneal muscle weakness. This pathoanatomy results in medial deviation and subluxation of the midfoot and hindfoot varus. The newborn's clubfoot is manipulated daily by a trained physical therapist to relax the posterior tibialis muscle and stretch the medial fibrous zone. Stretching is augmented with peroneal strengthening and taping. The medial tissues are stretched first, to correct the medial subluxation of the navicular. Forefoot adduction is corrected next by further stretching of the medial midfoot and forefoot. Simultaneous reduction of the forefoot adduction and hindfoot varus is then performed, followed by correction of the ankle equinus. After correction is obtained, serial taping with elastic tape is used to help maintain the position of the foot and ankle. Continuous passive motion with a specially designed machine has also been used as an adjunct to daily manipulations.[40] Daily stretching sessions are performed for the first 2 months of treatment, followed by formal physical therapy 3 times weekly until the patient is 6 months of age. Most of the correction is obtained by the age of 3 months, but daily stretching and taping is performed until stable correction is achieved and the patient is walking.

Surgery may be required when complete correction cannot be achieved through stretching and taping, or if relapse of the clubfoot occurs. The type and amount of surgery varies according to the need of the patient: patients with an isolated equinus contracture after stretches may require only an Achilles tenotomy, whereas patients with more pronounced residual deformity may require more extensive surgery, such as a posteromedial release. As should be evident from this intensive treatment program, parental participation and involvement are critical for success. The functional method, with its combination of stretching, continuous passive motion, and limited surgery, produces results rated as good to excellent in 60% to 80% of patients, and the rate of recurrence with this technique seems similar to that of the Ponseti method.[17,40,41]

Surgical treatment also continues to play a role in the treatment of clubfoot. Although the trend has been to move away from comprehensive subtalar releases and tendon lengthening, there are selected patients in whom surgery is required. Patients requiring surgical correction include those in whom the Ponseti technique has not worked or who have experienced relapses or patients who have club feet associated with syndromes or neurologic conditions.[36–38] Serial casting before surgical intervention may help achieve partial correction of the clubfoot, thereby making any subsequent surgery less extensive. The corrective surgery, instead of being a "one-size-fits-all" comprehensive release, can then be tailored to the specific deformity present in the foot. This approach, popularized by Bensahel as an "à la carte" release, releases and lengthens structures only as needed.[42] The procedure is tailored to correct the deformity that is present and typically involves tendon lengthening as well as releases of the posterior subtalar and ankle joints and the talonavicular joint.[42] This more limited approach views surgery as an adjunct to casting and attempts to minimize the scarring and risk of overcorrection that may occur with more aggressive procedures.

The treatment of clubfoot in older children, adolescents, and young adults is much less well defined. Good results with a modified Ponseti technique have been described in children with untreated clubfoot up to the age of 6 years.[30] In general, treatment needs to be individualized to address the various deformities that may be present. Common scenarios of recurrent or undercorrected clubfoot in older age groups include recurrent equinus deformity and recurrent cavovarus.

Recurrent equinus is a fairly common problem in older individuals with a clubfoot. Patients with equinus may present with poorly defined activity-related ankle, foot, or anterior knee pain. The onset is typically gradual, and in the skeletally immature patient, symptoms may be preceded by a rapid increase in height. Typically, the physical examination is significant for limited ankle dorsiflexion, as well as callosities on the plantar surface beneath the metatarsal heads. Initial treatment typically consists of stretches, which should include exercises to be performed at home, but formal physical therapy may be required as well. Patients with an equinus contracture resistant to nonoperative treatment should be considered for operative intervention. Before any surgery, careful preoperative analysis is required to accurately define the source of the plantar flexion. The plantar flexion may be from the ankle or from the midfoot. Accurate standing radiographs of the foot and ankle will help define the source of the deformity and aid in surgical planning. If the deformity is through the ankle joint and is the result of a contracture of the ankle joint and/or the gastrocnemius-soleus complex, correction can be achieved through a soft tissue procedure alone, such as an open lengthening of the Achilles tendon with a posterior ankle release. If the plantar flexion is occurring through the midfoot, a midfoot procedure such as a plantar release coupled with a midfoot extension osteotomy may be required for correction.

Recurrent cavovarus deformity occurring after operative clubfoot treatment may be secondary to dorsal rotary subluxation or dislocation of the navicular through the talonavicular joint.[43,44] This displacement of the navicular may be seen in patients who have had medial releases to correct their clubfoot: the medial border of the navicular rotates dorsally, effectively shortening the medial column of the foot and resulting in a cavovarus deformity of the foot. The subluxation or dislocation is recognized on plain radiographs, and the navicular may seem small and dysplastic. Rotary displacement of the navicular may be successfully treated with an open reduction of the talonavicular joint along with a talonavicular fusion.[44] This procedure may be combined with other procedures as required and seems to be effective in improving the position and appearance of the foot.

The patient with a residual or recurrent clubfoot who presents after multiple operative procedures presents one of the most challenging scenarios for the treating surgeon. A patient with a short, scarred, deformed foot may be best treated with gradual correction of the deformity with an external fixator.[45–48] A device capable of 3-dimensional correction should be used, and multiple deformities through the foot and ankle can be addressed simultaneously. Historically, this treatment has been hampered by high rates of recurrence.[45,48] Performing osteotomy before distraction, or arthrodesis after correction is obtained, may be of benefit in decreasing the recurrence rate after correction of clubfoot by gradual distraction.[45,46] This technique is highly demanding and has a high complication rate; it should be used only by surgeons who are experienced in external fixation and deformity correction.

SUMMARY

The incidence of clubfoot has remained remarkably constant through time. Its causes are still unknown, although strides are being made toward uncovering a genetic basis for the disease. The last decade has seen a seismic shift in the treatment of clubfoot, away from a universal operative approach toward a more nuanced approach involving manipulation and selective surgical intervention. Several nonoperative techniques have been developed and are now the standard of treatment throughout the world. Despite these improvements in clubfoot care, surgical treatments are still needed and beneficial in patients in whom the condition relapses or who do not completely respond to casting or stretching. The treatment of the neglected, residual, or relapsed clubfoot, however, remains a major challenge. Careful preoperative evaluation and surgical planning are needed to optimize results for this difficult problem.

REFERENCES

1. Dobbs MB, Gurnett CA. Update on clubfoot: etiology and treatment. Clin Orthop Relat Res 2009;467(5):1146–53.
2. Wynne-Davies R. Genetic and environmental factors in the etiology of talipes equinovarus. Clin Orthop Relat Res 1972;84:9–13.
3. Beals RK. Club foot in the Maori: a genetic study of 50 kindreds. N Z Med J 1978; 88(618):144–6.
4. Dunn PM. Congenital postural deformities: perinatal associations. Proc R Soc Med 1972;65(8):735–8.
5. Honein MA, Paulozzi LJ, Moore CA. Family history, maternal smoking, and clubfoot: an indication of a gene-environment interaction. Am J Epidemiol 2000; 152(7):658–65.
6. Hootnick DR, Levinsohn EM, Crider RJ, et al. Congenital arterial malformations associated with clubfoot. A report of two cases. Clin Orthop Relat Res 1982; 167:160–3.
7. Levinsohn EM, Hootnick DR, Packard DS Jr. Consistent arterial abnormalities associated with a variety of congenital malformations of the human lower limb. Invest Radiol 1991;26(4):364–73.
8. Sodre H, Bruschini S, Mestriner LA, et al. Arterial abnormalities in talipes equinovarus as assessed by angiography and the Doppler technique. J Pediatr Orthop 1990;10(1):101–4.
9. Dickinson KC, Meyer RE, Kotch J. Maternal smoking and the risk for clubfoot in infants. Birth Defects Res A Clin Mol Teratol 2008;82(2):86–91.
10. Karakurt L, Yilmaz E, Serin E, et al. Plasma total homocysteine level in mothers of children with clubfoot. J Pediatr Orthop 2003;23(5):658–60.
11. Lochmiller C, Johnston D, Scott A, et al. Genetic epidemiology study of idiopathic talipes equinovarus. Am J Med Genet 1998;79(2):90–6.

12. Dietz F. The genetics of idiopathic clubfoot. Clin Orthop Relat Res 2002;401: 39–48.
13. Herzenberg JE, Radler C, Bor N. Ponseti versus traditional methods of casting for idiopathic clubfoot. J Pediatr Orthop 2002;22(4):517–21.
14. Morcuende JA, Dolan LA, Dietz FR, et al. Radical reduction in the rate of extensive corrective surgery for clubfoot using the Ponseti method. Pediatrics 2004; 113(2):376–80.
15. Ponseti IV, Zhivkov M, Davis N, et al. Treatment of the complex idiopathic clubfoot. Clin Orthop Relat Res 2006;451:171–6.
16. Kite JH. Nonoperative treatment of congenital clubfoot. Clin Orthop Relat Res 1972;84:29–38.
17. Noonan KJ, Richards BS. Nonsurgical management of idiopathic clubfoot. J Am Acad Orthop Surg 2003;11(6):392–402.
18. Turco VJ. Surgical correction of the resistant club foot. One-stage posteromedial release with internal fixation: a preliminary report. J Bone Joint Surg Am 1971; 53(3):477–97.
19. Turco VJ. Resistant congenital club foot–one-stage posteromedial release with internal fixation. A follow-up report of a fifteen-year experience. J Bone Joint Surg Am 1979;61(6A):805–14.
20. McKay DW. New concept of and approach to clubfoot treatment: section I-principles and morbid anatomy. J Pediatr Orthop 1982;2(4):347–56.
21. Simons GW. Complete subtalar release in club feet. Part I–A preliminary report. J Bone Joint Surg Am 1985;67(7):1044–55.
22. Atar D, Lehman WB, Grant AD. Complications in clubfoot surgery. Orthop Rev 1991;20(3):233–9.
23. Dobbs MB, Nunley R, Schoenecker PL. Long-term follow-up of patients with clubfeet treated with extensive soft-tissue release. J Bone Joint Surg Am 2006;88(5): 986–96.
24. Ippolito E, Farsetti P, Caterini R, et al. Long-term comparative results in patients with congenital clubfoot treated with two different protocols. J Bone Joint Surg Am 2003;85(7):1286–94.
25. Ponseti IV. Treatment of congenital club foot. J Bone Joint Surg Am 1992;74(3): 448–54.
26. Ponseti IV, Morcuende JA. Current management of idiopathic clubfoot questionnaire: a multicenter study. J Pediatr Orthop 2004;24(4):448.
27. Dobbs MB, Rudzki JR, Purcell DB, et al. Factors predictive of outcome after use of the Ponseti method for the treatment of idiopathic clubfeet. J Bone Joint Surg Am 2004;86(1):22–7.
28. Coss HS, Hennrikus WL. Parent satisfaction comparing two bandage materials used during serial casting in infants. Foot Ankle Int 1996;17(8):483–6.
29. Pittner DE, Klingele KE, Beebe AC. Treatment of clubfoot with the Ponseti method: a comparison of casting materials. J Pediatr Orthop 2008;28(2):250–3.
30. Spiegel DA, Shrestha OP, Sitoula P, et al. Ponseti method for untreated idiopathic clubfeet in Nepalese patients from 1 to 6 years of age. Clin Orthop Relat Res 2009;467(5):1164–70.
31. Dobbs MB, Gordon JE, Walton T, et al. Bleeding complications following percutaneous tendoachilles tenotomy in the treatment of clubfoot deformity. J Pediatr Orthop 2004;24(4):353–7.
32. Parada SA, Baird GO, Auffant RA, et al. Safety of percutaneous tendoachilles tenotomy performed under general anesthesia on infants with idiopathic clubfoot. J Pediatr Orthop 2009;29(8):916–9.

33. Halanski MA, Davison JE, Huang JC, et al. Ponseti method compared with surgical treatment of clubfoot: a prospective comparison. J Bone Joint Surg Am 2010;92(2):270–8.
34. Lehman WB, Mohaideen A, Madan S, et al. A method for the early evaluation of the Ponseti (Iowa) technique for the treatment of idiopathic clubfoot. J Pediatr Orthop B 2003;12(2):133–40.
35. Cooper DM, Dietz FR. Treatment of idiopathic clubfoot. A thirty-year follow-up note. J Bone Joint Surg Am 1995;77(10):1477–89.
36. Boehm S, Limpaphayom N, Alaee F, et al. Early results of the Ponseti method for the treatment of clubfoot in distal arthrogryposis. J Bone Joint Surg Am 2008; 90(7):1501–7.
37. Gerlach DJ, Gurnett CA, Limpaphayom N, et al. Early results of the Ponseti method for the treatment of clubfoot associated with myelomeningocele. J Bone Joint Surg Am 2009;91(6):1350–9.
38. van Bosse HJ, Marangoz S, Lehman WB, et al. Correction of arthrogrypotic club-foot with a modified Ponseti technique. Clin Orthop Relat Res 2009;467(5): 1283–93.
39. Bensahel H, Guillaume A, Czukonyi Z, et al. Results of physical therapy for idio-pathic clubfoot: a long-term follow-up study. J Pediatr Orthop 1990;10(2):189–92.
40. Dimeglio A, Bonnet F, Mazeau P, et al. Orthopaedic treatment and passive motion machine: consequences for the surgical treatment of clubfoot. J Pediatr Orthop B 1996;5(3):173–80.
41. Richards BS, Faulks S, Rathjen KE, et al. A comparison of two nonoperative methods of idiopathic clubfoot correction: the Ponseti method and the French functional (physiotherapy) method. J Bone Joint Surg Am 2008;90(11):2313–21.
42. Bensahel H, Csukonyi Z, Desgrippes Y, et al. Surgery in residual clubfoot: one-stage medioposterior release "a la carte". J Pediatr Orthop 1987;7(2):145–8.
43. Kuo KN, Jansen LD. Rotatory dorsal subluxation of the navicular: a complication of clubfoot surgery. J Pediatr Orthop 1998;18(6):770–4.
44. Swaroop VT, Wenger DR, Mubarak SJ. Talonavicular fusion for dorsal subluxation of the navicular in resistant clubfoot. Clin Orthop Relat Res 2009;467(5):1314–8.
45. Burns JK, Sullivan R. Correction of severe residual clubfoot deformity in adoles-cents with the Ilizarov technique. Foot Ankle Clin 2004;9(3):571–82, ix.
46. El-Mowafi H, El-Alfy B, Refai M. Functional outcome of salvage of residual and recurrent deformities of clubfoot with Ilizarov technique. Foot Ankle Surg 2009; 15(1):3–6.
47. Ferreira RC, Costa MT. Recurrent clubfoot–approach and treatment with external fixation. Foot Ankle Clin 2009;14(3):435–45.
48. Freedman JA, Watts H, Otsuka NY. The Ilizarov method for the treatment of resis-tant clubfoot: is it an effective solution? J Pediatr Orthop 2006;26(4):432–7.

Residual Clubfoot in Children

Michael G. Uglow, FRCS(Tr&Orth)*,
Harish V. Kurup, MS(Orth), FRCS(Orth)

KEYWORDS

• Residual • Clubfoot • Deformity • Surgery

The treatment of children who have clubfeet has been revolutionized with the belated acceptance of Ponseti's method of serial stretching and casting. The improved results from nonoperative treatment have greatly reduced the need for early surgical correction of clubfoot, and rates of surgery have decreased tremendously in recent years to as low as 2.5% in the best hands.[1] Most doctors who have a significant practice of treating clubfeet will have two groups of patients: those treated with Ponseti's method and those from preceding years who were managed surgically. Additionally, there are two broad groups, the idiopathic clubfeet and those that are deemed to be complex, either because of teratologic or neurologic etiology.

Each group of patients has a similar presentation, but different treatment options may be required depending on the etiology and previous treatment. Despite best efforts, some feet remain recalcitrant to treatment and residual deformities do occur. This article discusses the deformities that can present and the treatment options.

The challenge in treating clubfeet is to provide children who have a functional plantigrade foot. After the treatment of primary and recurrent deformity, residual deformity may be present, not all of which will cause functional deficit. The treating physician must decide what is relevant and can be improved and what has no influence on function or symptoms. As with all treatment decisions, attending surgeons must decide whether they have a realistic opportunity to improve function for the child and reduce symptoms. The appearance of the foot is important, but only when pain and function have been assessed. Any intervention must address these two factors first. Often appearance also will improve, but treatment priority must be identified.

Recurrence of the deformities associated with idiopathic clubfoot occurs in 20% to 30% of patients, and continued follow-up of children who have clubfeet is essential to identify and treat recurrences expeditiously. Even after successful conservative treatment, 2% to 20% may still require surgical procedures to correct residual deformities.[2] Long-term studies evaluating patient function show that the outcome is not exclusively dependent on anatomic considerations. Ippolito and colleagues[3] followed two groups

Department of Paediatric Orthopaedics, Southampton University Hospital, Tremona Road, Southampton, Hampshire, SO16 6YD, UK
* Corresponding author.
E-mail address: m.uglow@btclick.com

Foot Ankle Clin N Am 15 (2010) 245–264
doi:10.1016/j.fcl.2010.01.003
foot.theclinics.com

of patients into their 20s and found that limited posterior release had better results than extensive releases in combination with conservative treatment. Early comprehensive surgical release is still necessary in treating clubfoot in special circumstances such as arthrogryposis.

PATHOANATOMY

In congenital clubfoot, genetic factors and intrauterine packaging have been deemed responsible for the deformities, as have neuromuscular conditions. Most cases have no identifiable cause and are labeled *idiopathic*. The deformity in clubfoot is complex and involves the ankle and subtalar and midtarsal joints. The forefoot is invariably affected, usually through relative shortening of the long flexor tendons, and is certainly influenced during treatment if this imbalance is not addressed.

Equinus deformity is present at the ankle, and internal rotation, inversion, and adduction deformity at the subtalar joint. This combined inversion and adduction deformity occurs in unison because of the oblique configuration of the subtalar joint axis and is referred to as hindfoot varus. The talus and calcaneus have inherently abnormal anatomy in clubfoot, and the calcaneus is also internally rotated beneath the talus. At the mid-tarsal joint, the forefoot is adducted and plantar flexed in relation to the hindfoot, and the plantar fascia contributes to this. The tarsal bones develop secondary adaptive changes in longstanding cases, as seen in those that remain untreated[4] and those with residual deformity.

Underlying abnormalities that contribute to these deformities are both soft tissue and bony. Soft tissue abnormalities affecting the hindfoot are contractures of the gastrocsoleus, tibialis posterior, the peroneal sheath, and tendons. Other soft tissue contractures, such as joint capsules and ligaments, develop subsequently and affect most structures on the medial and posterior aspects of the foot and ankle. Pirani and colleagues[5] studied MRI scanning in patients undergoing the Ponseti method and have shown that early institution of conservative treatment helps by stretching the soft tissues and allowing adaptive bony changes to overcome these deformities.

Late residual deformities after clubfoot treatment can be dynamic, stiff, or rigid and may affect each part of the foot and ankle. Equinus, varus, and internal rotation of the calcaneum, and true equinus of the ankle are common.

In surgically treated feet, overcorrection results in calcaneus and valgus deformity of the hindfoot. In the mid- and forefoot, supination and adduction deformities are the most common problems encountered, but overcorrection resulting in a midfoot break also may be seen, and has a higher incidence in patients who have ligamentous hyperlaxity. Subluxation of the navicular may also be present, invariably associated with talar head and neck deformity. Dorsal bunion of the metatarsophalangeal joints is primarily caused by soft tissue contracture on the plantar surface with shortening of the long flexors, but an assessment of the metatarsal anatomy is paramount to effective treatment.

Patients who have unilateral clubfoot may develop limb and foot length discrepancy by the completion of growth. In operatively treated clubfeet, Docquier and colleagues[2] found a mean limb length discrepancy of 13 mm (8-20 mm) and foot length discrepancy of 15 mm (5–29 mm). The mean calf diameter discrepancy was 43 mm (15–60 mm). Slanting of the posterior part of distal tibial articular surface was noted in 28% cases, and was seen exclusively in cases that had Achilles lengthening without posterior capsular release. The same finding was observed by Ponseti and colleagues,[6] and this results in a decreased tibiotalar angle that contributes to the cavus deformity.

Experts have suggested that this may be preventable with posterior capsulotomy in addition to Achilles tenotomy.[2]

Medial tibial torsion has proved to be a controversial topic, but more recent studies consider it no longer relevant.[2,4] A derotation osteotomy in the distal tibial metaphysis can be used to treat internal rotation deformity of the hindfoot when there are good reasons to avoid surgery on the foot, despite whether a rotation in the tibia itself is present.

Notching of the anterior lip of the distal tibial epiphysis was seen in 63% of patients in the series by Ponseti and colleagues[6] and 52% in that by Docquier and colleagues.[2] This effect was caused by the pressure of the talar head during foot dorsiflexion, leading to bone growth arrest. In normal feet, no contact occurs between the talar head and the tibial epiphysis during dorsiflexion, but preventing this growth arrest is impossible in clubfeet because of a shortened talus.[2]

The talar and calcaneal lengths are significantly smaller in clubfeet in utero, which persists regardless of intervention and restricts ankle movements as the anterior lip of the tibial epiphysis projects to or beyond the level of the head of the talus. The height of the talar trochlea in clubfeet is always smaller than in normal feet, denoting a flat-top talus that decreases ankle joint congruency and mobility, as shown with dynamic views. Clubfoot deformity is important to correct before walking age to prevent severe talar flattening.[2] The range of ankle dorsiflexion and subtalar and midtarsal joint motion is restricted in clubfeet compared with the normal opposite side.[6]

Avascular necrosis of the talus is a serious potential complication of clubfoot surgery. Cummings and colleagues[7] have shown that absence of growth lines in the talus during follow-up is predictive of future collapse, which may lead to flattening of the head of talus or hypoplasia of the talar head and neck. Many of the more severe feet have an impaired vascular supply and are vulnerable to increased forces and the effects of surgery.[8] Combined one-stage medial and lateral release has been shown to increase the incidence of vascular insult to the talus,[9] whereas Uglow and Clarke[10] found a two-stage release to be safe.

Docquier and colleagues[2] showed that the navicular developed wedging in 28% of patients, medial subluxation in 56%, and dorsal subluxation in 48% after surgical treatment. This effect can be attributed to an overactive tibialis anterior tendon and midfoot hypermobility. A slight residual metatarsal adduction is common and rarely causes any symptoms or functional deficit. Cavus usually affects plantar flexion of only the first metatarsal, but the entire midfoot can be involved. Overactivity of the tibialis anterior contributes to the elevation of the base of the first ray but causes supination of the forefoot more commonly than pure cavus. Initially, the deformity is dynamic and presents an ideal opportunity for intervention before secondary changes occur, which is an important principle in the management of residual deformity, because the outcome of all deformities will invariably have a better outcome if treatment is initiated before deformities become stiff and secondary changes occur.

ETIOLOGY AND THE EFFECT OF DEFORMITIES
Residual Equinus

Residual equinus or equinovarus is not uncommon after surgical or nonsurgical treatment of clubfoot (**Fig. 1**).[11] Early Achilles tenotomy, as used in the Ponseti technique, reduces the incidence of residual equinus deformity but may lead to excessive ankle dorsiflexion.[12] Not all children treated with the Ponseti method require a tenotomy of the Achilles, and it should be withheld if the equinus deformity corrects completely. Scher and colleagues[13] report a 72% rate of Achilles tenotomy, similar to this article's senior author's experience of 70%.[14]

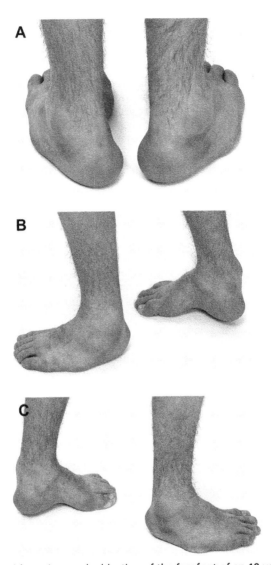

Fig. 1. Heel varus with equinus and adduction of the forefoot of an 18-year-old man's feet. The large prominences laterally show clearly the main load-bearing areas. The previous scarring can be seen medially and on the lateral aspect of the heels. (*A*) Rear view. (*B*) Left-side view. (*C*) Right-side view.

The need for tenotomy is predictably higher in grade IV feet according to Diméglio and colleagues classification,[15] and in feet with a Pirani score of 5.0 or higher.[16] The correction achieved is full dorsiflexion at the end of treatment, despite the need for a tenotomy. However, ongoing functional assessment is being studied to ensure that relapse and recurrent deformity remains minimal and to ensure that no increase in late equinus deformity occurs that could be attributable to not performing a tenotomy. Alvarez and colleagues[17] used Botox injections as an alternative to Achilles tenotomy and reported that the overall surgical rate for residual deformities reduced to 15.4% after 5 years follow-up.

For children who have increasing equinus, the heel begins to lift off the floor, which may result in the absence of heel strike during the stance phase of gait and increase the time that the forefoot is loaded. Calluses can form under the metatarsal heads and pain can occur in the midfoot or present as metatarsalgia. The more flexible the foot the better the function, but if excessive equinus occurs, excessive compensatory dorsiflexion may occur across the midfoot joints. A more common adaptive change is for hyperextension to occur at the knee, the so-called back knee gait. For normal gait to occur, the knee must propel forward beyond the mid-axis of the ankle in the sagittal plane, which requires the ankle to dorsiflex. In clubfoot, equinus of the talus is common and this frequently interferes with gait. In the presence of equinus, when the foot is placed flat to the floor the tibia is inclined and the knee must hyperextend to compensate.[18] These mechanics can contribute to symptoms, especially as children become older and less flexible.

Residual Heel Varus

Residual heel varus (see **Fig. 1**) can be present in varying degrees and has been reported to affect 10%[19] to 80%[2] of mature patients treated for clubfoot. This condition can occur from either inadequate initial correction, recurrence, or a combination of these. Determining whether the deformity contributes to symptoms is important in planning a correction strategy. Most patients have residual varus of less than 10° and this is well tolerated. Occasionally the heel pad is mobile and the apparent degree of varus can be exaggerated, and therefore patients must be examined carefully to assess true bony varus.

Residual Cavus

Residual cavus is also seen commonly after clubfoot treatment,[20] caused by a tight plantar fascia, an overactive tibialis anterior, and dorsal subluxation of the navicular. As with all cavus deformities, whether only the first ray is depressed or the entire forefoot is involved must be determined. Mosca[21] also highlighted the importance of the peroneus longus in the depression of the first ray, but this is not felt to be a significant factor in idiopathic clubfoot.

Dynamic Supination

Dynamic supination is the most common deformity seen after conservative or surgical treatment of clubfoot.[22] This deformity results from a strong tibialis anterior with weak antagonists. Why the tibialis anterior maintains normal function, when other muscles do not, is unknown. This condition can also contribute to cavus, varus, and adduction deformities. It causes functional problems, such as inability to maintain the foot plantigrade during walking and increased shoe wear. If dynamic supination remains, then progression to a fixed deformity is virtually inevitable (**Fig. 2**). Early treatment should be encouraged when soft tissue surgery alone may afford full correction.

Forefoot Adduction

Residual forefoot adduction is caused by an overacting tibialis anterior, medial displacement of the navicular on the talar head, and residual medial deviation of the talar neck and head (**Fig. 3**). Although medial displacement of the navicular is widely believed to be the underlying deformity, Wallander and colleagues[23] found no correlation between residual forefoot adduction and navicular position according to ultrasound. True metatarsus varus also contributes to the residual adduction in many patients.[24]

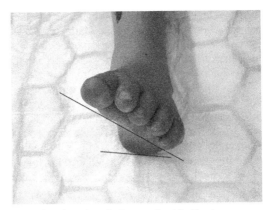

Fig. 2. Supination of the forefoot in relation to the hindfoot.

Intoeing Gait

Intoeing gait is caused by residual forefoot adduction and dynamic supination deformities in most cases. Patients who have idiopathic clubfoot (including unilateral cases) also have been shown to have increased hip internal rotation, suggesting an exaggerated femoral anteversion.[25] Gait analysis can be helpful in assessing proximal deformities in children who have residual clubfoot before corrective surgery is performed.[26]

Overcorrection

Overcorrection of deformities resulting in a flatfoot is a recognized complication, especially in open surgical release.[27] The risk is significantly higher in children who have generalized joint laxity. This complication was historically attributed to division of the talocalcaneal interosseous ligament, but El-Deeb and colleagues[28] found no association after a prospective comparative study in 66 feet followed up for a mean of 28 months.

Rotary Subluxation of Navicular

Rotary subluxation of the navicular has been reported in as many as 7.1% cases after surgical release.[29] Anatomic models suggest that the medial border of the navicular

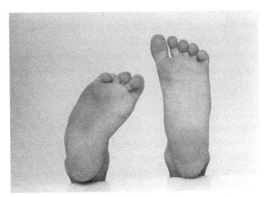

Fig. 3. Residual forefoot adduction. Note the bean-shaped right foot and relative length of the longer lateral and shorter medial columns.

rotates superiorly in the coronal plane and mimics a dorsal subluxation, which can lead to a cavovarus deformity and contributes to medial column shortening with resultant pain, gait problems, and increased shoe wear. The navicular is invariably dysmorphic, being more triangular in profile, and reflects the overall shape of the mid- and forefoot based on the position of the apex. Talonavicular pain may occur from degeneration of the joint as age advances. Three-dimensional imaging with CT scanning can be helpful in understanding the navicular's true shape and identifying any degenerative changes.

Dorsal Bunion

Iatrogenic dorsal bunion can be seen after surgery for clubfoot,[30] and arises from elevation of the first metatarsal head from overactivity of the tibialis anterior and flexor hallucis longus,[11] plantar flexion contracture at the first metatarsophalangeal joint, and dorsiflexion contracture of the tarsometatarsal joint.[31]

EVALUATION
Clinical

Clinical examination includes assessment of flexibility and static deformities, the correction achievable, and range of motion of individual joints. Dynamic supination can be easily recognized on simple observation of gait. Rotational profile of the limb must be assessed and is well described by Staheli and colleagues[32] using foot progression angle, hip rotation, thigh–foot angle, and transmalleolar axis. Laaveg and Ponseti[33] described a scale popular for assessing function and patient satisfaction in residual clubfoot, which takes into account patient satisfaction, function, position of heel, passive motion, and gait. Assessment of skin quality, particularly in relation to previous scars and grafts, is essential along with examination of the vascular supply. These factors may influence if a deformity can be corrected acutely or whether staged procedures are needed to prevent excessive swelling and the consequent complications affecting the soft tissues and vascular supply.

Radiographs

To optimize the radiographic studies, the foot should be held in the position of best correction.[34] Weight-bearing anteroposterior radiographs of the ankle and weight-bearing lateral radiographs of the foot and ankle are a good starting point (**Fig. 4**). The X-ray beam should be focused on the hindfoot, approximately 30° from the vertical for the anteroposterior radiograph, and the lateral radiograph should be transmalleolar with the fibula overlapping the posterior half of the tibia to avoid rotational distortion. The talocalcaneal angle and talar–first metatarsal angle are measured on anteroposterior and lateral radiographs.[34] Dynamic views in maximal plantar and dorsiflexion can be used to measure the mobility in the ankle joint compared with the midfoot.[2] Heel alignment should be assessed using a longitudinal view of the long axis of the calcaneus to the tibia using Saltzman and el-Khoury[35] modification of the Cobey view. Limb length can be assessed with limb-length measurement radiographs in unilateral cases and to identify longitudinal angular deformities at the ankle and knee joint. Weight-bearing digital length films with a mobile tube remaining perpendicular to the long axis of the limb (microdose digital scanography) is preferred, but orthoroentgenograms are reliable.

Computed Tomography Scan

Computed tomography (CT) scan can be useful in assessing bony and joint deformities, and modern software provides the ability to produce three-dimensional

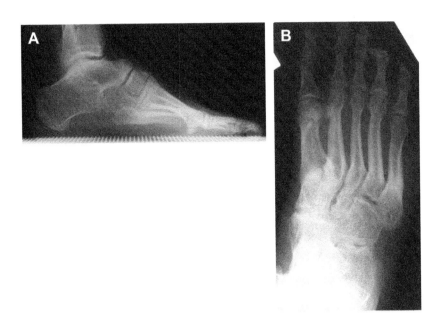

Fig. 4. Radiographs of a 30-year-old man who previously underwent subtalar and talonavicular fusion for painful degeneration secondary to clubfoot. (*A*) A lateral weight-bearing radiograph. Note the dysmorphic and flattened talus, the plantar flexed first ray, and the stress changes in the fifth metatarsal from overloading. Irregular margins of the calcaneal cuboid joint can also be seen. (*B*) A weight-bearing oblique view. Note the relative shortening of the fist metatarsal from the plantar flexed position, the stress changes of the fourth and fifth metatarsals, and the irregularity of the calcaneal cuboid articulation. This joint is not yet painful, and avoiding fusion to retain some motion is worthwhile.

images.[36] Feet should be held in neutral position by a radiolucent support or splint. Three-dimensional reconstructions can allow better appreciation of deformities and relationship between individual bones. Cross-sectional imaging is useful in assessing the presence of degenerative changes of the joints. The treating surgeon should decide whether the benefit of the additional information obtained with CT outweighs the higher-than-usual radiation dose needed for each individual case.

Gait Analysis

When doubt exists or proximal problems are suspected, gait analysis can be useful in assessment. This assessment typically includes computerized motion analysis and dynamic electromyography. Footswitches with pressure sensors under the heel, first and fifth metatarsal heads, and great toe can be used to determine the phasing of muscle activity and detect the presence of forefoot pronation or supination. This technique can also detect subtle abnormalities, such as tibial torsion, which contributes to the deformity. Quantitative gait analysis changed the choice of procedure in 63% of cases in one study involving 35 patients,[26] but for most cases simple observational analysis in the clinic setting should suffice. Formal analysis is useful as a research tool, but will be discussed further in a separate article.

Pedobarography

Dynamic measurement of the pressure distribution on the bottom of the foot through all stages of the gait cycle is useful in assessing the maximum force, contact area, and peak pressure in clubfeet. Most children who have treated clubfeet show reduced peak pressure over the medial hindfoot and forefoot, with increased pressure over the lateral midfoot despite good functional outcome.[37] This assessment can be useful in detecting subtle dynamic supination but is unlikely to influence surgical decision making.

Joint Injections

In patients who may have degeneration, the clinical and radiographic findings do not necessarily correlate well. Local anesthetic injections into specific joints can be very helpful in determining which joints are contributing to symptoms. If fusions are required, this approach will ensure that asymptomatic joints can be left alone and only symptomatic ones are fused.

TREATMENT

Residual clubfoot deformities can be managed with nonoperative treatment, soft tissue procedures, osteotomies, or fusion. Individual deformities are considered and treatment discussed accordingly. Despite anatomic deformities, many patients can have satisfactory function and may not need corrective surgery.

The treating surgeon must have a thorough understanding of the individual deformities and the deforming forces involved. An à la carte approach is necessary to treat each abnormality on its merit always with an appreciation of the resultant effect on the whole foot. One procedure in isolation rarely corrects the residual clubfoot. All factors must be carefully evaluated before a reconstructive program is initiated, starting proximally and working progressively and sequentially in a distal direction (**Fig. 5**). In principle, a philosophy of extra-articular osteotomies in combination with soft tissue rebalancing should be adopted, reserving fusion for symptomatic degeneration. If osteotomies are to be performed on more than one region of the foot, then staging them 2 weeks apart is wise to avoid complications from excessive swelling.

Residual Equinus

Conservative treatment of residual equinus includes manual stretching under anesthetic and casting or daily stretching program. Although some authors have claimed good success with stretching,[38] recurrence rates are generally considered to be high.

Achilles tenotomy or lengthening with or without posterior ankle capsulotomy is the most commonly used technique for residual equinus deformity. Equinus in older children presenting with clubfoot after 1 year of age can be successfully treated with Achilles tenotomy and Ponseti casting[39]; but as age increases, the chance that equinus can be adequately corrected by stretching alone decreases. Similarly, releasing the Achilles tendon to find no appreciable improvement in equinus position can be disappointing. The posterior ankle release must be added in younger patients and can be very effective, but as age increases the degree of correction is invariably less and recurrent scarring and contracture may occur, negating any gains in the longer term. Achilles lengthening can cause as much as a 23% decrease in plantar flexion power in surgically treated clubfeet.[40]

Limited soft tissue release followed by gradual correction using the Ilizarov ring fixator has shown good results in the management of resistant and neglected clubfeet.[41] The principle of tissue neogenesis rather than acute correction and subsequent fibrosis is appealing, especially for stiffer and syndromic feet. The appropriate age at which to stop performing posterior ankle release is difficult to determine, but the morphology of the talus must be assessed first to ensure that correction is not being blocked by bony deformity.

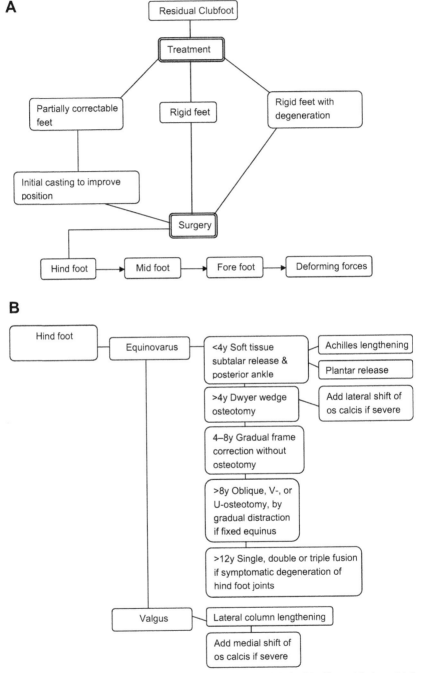

Fig. 5. Algorithms of treatment for (*A*) residual clubfoot, (*B*) the hindfoot, (*C*) the mid-foot, (*D*) the forefoot, and (*E*) the deforming forces.

C

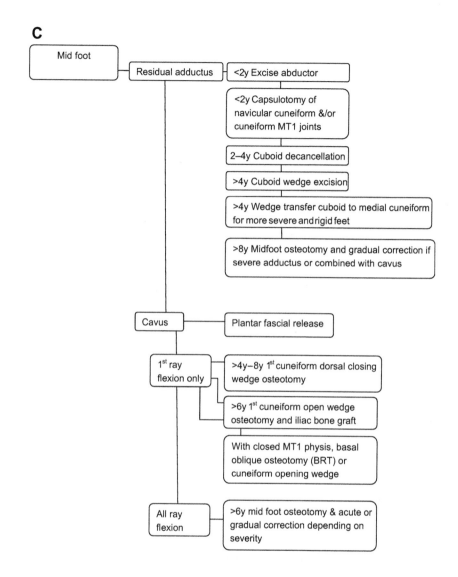

Fig. 5. (*continued*)

Swann and colleagues[4] observed that even though the calcaneum is in equinus, the talus is already fully dorsiflexed and lying in an abnormal position within the ankle mortise, which contributes to the failure of soft tissue procedures in residual equinus. He suggested anterior closing wedge osteotomy of the distal tibia in this situation. The authors were unable to find any published results on this technique.

Residual Heel Varus

Residual heel varus can be corrected only with calcaneal osteotomy or corrective fusion of the subtalar joint. The classical operation of medial opening wedge osteotomy of the calcaneum has been credited to Dwyer by Kumar and colleagues[42] and has shown very good results in long-term follow-up of up to 27 years, but medial

D

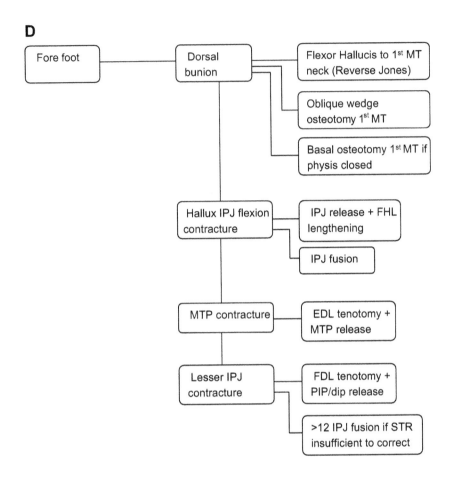

Fig. 5. (continued)

wound healing has been a major problem. A lateral closing wedge procedure is therefore preferred and, although the heel height is not increased as with the medial procedure, wound healing is much more reliable. Dwyer[43] also described this lateral procedure but did so for the treatment of pes cavus, although it is very reliable for treating residual heel varus in clubfoot. He believed that other deformities correct themselves once the heel is corrected, but experts now know that this is not true and that each individual component of the deformity must be addressed.

More versatile osteotomies have been described that offer simultaneous correction of deformities in different planes. The V-osteotomy[44] and U-osteotomy (or scythe-shaped osteotomy)[45] are similar in concept and followed by use of a frame for gradual correction of the deformity. These approaches allow correction of equinus, calcaneus, varus, valgus, and foot height as needed.

Residual Cavus

Residual cavus deformity can be corrected satisfactorily with a plantar release and serial casting,[46] the recurrence rates may be high, especially with advancing age. An assessment must be made as to whether the deformity affects the first ray or entire

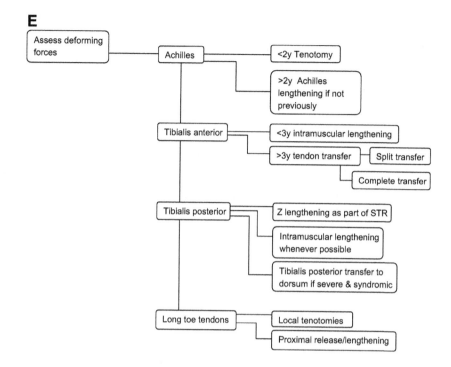

E

Assess deforming forces

- Achilles
  - <2y Tenotomy
  - >2y Achilles lengthening if not previously
- Tibialis anterior
  - <3y intramuscular lengthening
  - >3y tendon transfer
    - Split transfer
    - Complete transfer
- Tibialis posterior
  - Z lengthening as part of STR
  - Intramuscular lengthening whenever possible
  - Tibialis posterior transfer to dorsum if severe & syndromic
- Long toe tendons
  - Local tenotomies
  - Proximal release/lengthening

Fig. 5. (*continued*)

mid-foot. If only the first ray is involved, then, because the apex of the deformity is the medial cuneiform, the ideal choice of correction is an osteotomy of this bone and either a closing dorsal wedge or opening plantar wedge.[21,47] The choice is dependent on the flexibility of the ray. The closing wedge osteotomy is preferred because it removes the added morbidity of an iliac bone graft. However, increasing age decreases the possibility of a closing wedge, and the insertion of iliac bone graft as an opening wedge with the base into the plantar aspect of the medial cuneiform is reliable. The base can be rotated toward the medial aspect to aid correction of adductus if present. The graft may require securing with two smooth wires for 6 weeks, although the original description does not involve fixation.

In older children, the morbidity of the cuneiform procedure with graft can be avoided by operating on the first metatarsal using the oblique wedge osteotomy described by Barouk, Rippstein, and Toullec: the BRT osteotomy.[48] This procedure uses an osteotomy in the approximate plane of the sole of the foot and, as long as the plantar cortex is maintained, provides excellent stability and a large surface area for union. Internal fixation with low profile or headless screws is required.

The mid-foot V-osteotomy was originally described by Japas[49] for correcting cavus deformity from neurologic causes. This procedure offers correction of cavus only and therefore was adapted for clubfoot management as the Akron midtarsal dome osteotomy,[50] offering three-dimensional correction, including residual adduction. This technique is recommended for children older than 8 years but is technically difficult and requires considerable exposure and consequent risk to the soft tissues. A safer procedure is a straight osteotomy through a percutaneous approach using four 1-cm incisions along the cuneiform–cuboid axis.[51] Incisions are dorsomedial, dorsolateral, plantar lateral, and plantar medial, and a Gigli saw is threaded extraperiosteally from lateral to medial on the plantar surface and then onto the dorsal surface medially, and finally delivered through the dorsolateral incision. Paley and Tetsworth[51] states that the procedure can also be performed from medial to lateral. Placing two long smooth wires on either side of the intended site of osteotomy will ensure accurate passage of the Gigli saw. Modest corrections can be made acutely, but in severe deformities the same osteotomy can be used for gradual correction in a frame.

Dynamic Supination

Residual dynamic supination deformity is the most common sequel after surgical or nonsurgical treatment of clubfoot. Nonoperative treatment has little role in the management of this problem. Once the foot begins to show evidence of supination, it will not resolve and treatment will be required. The preferred procedure is a transfer of the tibialis anterior tendon, but in very young patients an intramuscular lengthening may be performed if intervention is required before the cuneiforms have ossified sufficiently. Dietz expressed concern in transferring a tendon into cartilage before the ossific nucleus is present, but the author are not aware of any studies examining this particular point (Dietz, personal communication, 2003).

Tendon has been shown to heal to cartilage earlier than to bone in a rabbit partial patellectomy model, but the difference diminishes as the healing process matures between 8 and 16 weeks. This finding supports adequate healing in the immature cuneiform but does not show whether growth is impaired.[52] An intramuscular lengthening is a safe procedure and may at best obviate the need for future transfer, or at least delay its requirement until the foot is more mature.[53]

Garceau[54] first described anterior tibial tendon transposition in 1940. The current techniques include transfer of the entire tendon either subcutaneously beneath the extensor retinaculum, above the retinaculum to the dorsum or lateral aspect of the mid-foot, or through a split tibialis anterior tendon transfer.[22] Thompson and colleagues[22] reported 88% good results in 137 feet with a minimum follow-up of 2 years. Concurrent additional procedures for other deformities did not affect the outcome.

Most authors agree that tibialis anterior transfer is effective in restoring muscle balance in residual clubfoot. The foot should be passively correctable to neutral before considering transfer of the tendon, and it can be combined with a revision procedure to correct residual fixed deformity if required.

Forefoot Adduction

Several procedures are described for treating residual adduction of the forefoot. Often the mid-foot has some flexibility and initial casting is recommended to improve the deformity, which reduces the extent of surgical intervention required. No fixed protocol exists for casting in cases of residual deformity, but weekly or bi-weekly cast changes should be attempted. Surgeons will be able to determine whether the deformity is improving or if it remains static, at which point surgery is performed to correct the remaining deformity.

Cumming and colleagues notes that residual forefoot adduction, if flexible, is corrected after tibialis anterior transfer in most patients when operated early. Isolated forefoot adduction in children younger than 2 years can be corrected through repeat soft tissue release.[34] In patients younger than 4 years, cuboid decancellation preserves the joint while shortening the lateral column.[34]

Rigid deformities at older ages require osteotomies for full correction. This procedure can involve opening wedge osteotomy of the medial cuneiform,[55] lateral closing wedge osteotomy of the cuboid,[56] or a combined procedure in which the wedge taken from the cuboid is transferred to the medial cuneiform.[57] From a technical standpoint, the medial osteotomy must include all the cuneiforms so that the point of correction is in the central part of the foot.

The original Dillwyn Evans[58] procedure used calcaneocuboid fusion to maintain correction but should ideally be reserved for older children because it decreases further growth of the lateral column. Lichtblau[59] describes a procedure to excise the distal calcaneus and preserve the cartilage of the cuboid, thus producing a pseudarthrosis with more chance for movement, at least theoretically. Significant stiffness has been found in longer-term follow-up of patients who underwent this procedure,[60] but only in more severe feet, and therefore determining whether the condition or the procedure is the main causative factor remains a challenge.

Intoeing Gait

Intoeing gait is corrected depending on the primary pathology, whether it is caused by dynamic supination or residual adduction. Any rotational deformity proximally in the tibia or femur are assessed and managed on its own merit. Supramalleolar osteotomies can be combined with posterior angulation to correct equinus concurrently.[34]

Overcorrection

Overcorrection after initial deformity correction results in a plano-valgus foot. The subtalar joint is usually stiff and the deformity rigid. Calcaneal lengthening is not preferred in the presence of subtalar stiffness, but if reducibility around the midfoot is possible, this procedure can correct the overcorrection.[61] In patients who have midfoot rigidity, medial translational osteotomy of the calcaneal tuberosity was suggested as a good salvage option (**Fig. 6**).[11] Plantar displacement of the calcaneal fragment can be performed to create an arch of the foot at the same time. The presence of ankle valgus contributing to the deformity should be assessed with weight-bearing radiographs and, if present, can be managed with eight-plate hemiepiphyseodesis of the medial side.[62]

Rotary Subluxation of Navicular

Dorsal rotary subluxation of navicular is a challenging problem and may cause significant symptoms in the midfoot. It does not usually respond to soft tissue procedures in older patients,[29] but reduction of the navicular through medial capsular release should

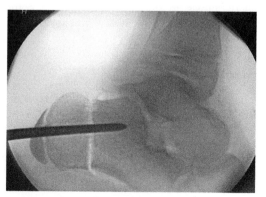

Fig. 6. Lateral image intensifier radiograph taken perioperatively showing a vertical calcaneal medialization osteotomy, stabilized with smooth wires.

be attempted in younger patients. In addition, the calcaneocuboid joint axis likely will also need to be addressed with soft tissue surgery. Talonavicular fusion has shown good short-term results,[63] but long-term outcome remains to be seen. For symptomatic older patients, fusion is the most reliable way to achieve reduction and gain adequate function.

Dorsal Bunion

A reverse Jones transfer, which involves transfer of the distal end of the flexor hallucis longus to the neck of the first metatarsal head through a drill-hole, has shown good results for dorsal bunions.[31] In patients who have a stiff tarsometatarsal joint, a proximal first metatarsal plantar flexion osteotomy will be required, but the physis at the base of the metatarsal is at risk until its closure. To accommodate the physis, the osteotomy must be performed more distally; an oblique wedge osteotomy provides good correction with little bone removal (the reverse BRT). The osteotomy is in the plane of the sole and can be fixed with headless screws to avoid need for removal. If tibialis anterior transfer was not performed previously, it may be performed because it has been shown to contribute to the development of the dorsal bunion and elevation of the first metatarsal.

Lesser Toes

The toes must be addressed last, after the hind- and mid-foot are corrected. If multiple procedures are required, staging the operations may allow a reduction in swelling and make the procedures safer. The most common deformities encountered are flexion contractures of the metatarsophalangeal and interphalangeal joints from the relative shortening of the flexor tendons. Initial release of the tendons may allow correction if the joints are correctable, but with increasing age the joints are more likely to be contracted and capsular releases will be required to achieve correction. Proximal intramuscular lengthening as part of a soft tissue release is a good option to reduce the risk for local scar adhesion in the toes, but if significant scarring is present along the course of the tendons, a proximal lengthening will not be sufficient and tenotomies distally will be necessary.

A step-wise approach is advisable, dealing first with the tendon and proceeding to release the joint, which usually requires division of the collateral ligaments and release of the plantar plate. In adolescents, a fusion of the interphalangeal joint may be necessary because the digit may need to be shortened to allow full correction. In this case, a condylectomy at the proximal joint surface, but leaving the distal articular surface intact, allows a pseudarthrosis to develop rather than a complete fusion. This approach will not lead to recurrence, because the flexor tendon will already have been divided.

COMBINED CORRECTION OF DEFORMITIES

The à la carte approach requires assessment of all deformities of the foot and their relation to each other. Treatment inevitably involves multiple separate procedures to achieve correction and result in a plantigrade foot. With increasing complexity and stiffness, especially in the presence of poorer soft tissues and vascular supply, performing multiple procedures is associated with increasing risks related to swelling and wound healing. Staging procedures is often wise and, although this can lead to scheduling pressures, is seldom regretted.

The Ilizarov apparatus has been combined with various osteotomies to provide distraction osteogenesis for the correction of residual deformities in the residual clubfoot. Equinus, varus of the hindfoot, midfoot adductus, and cavus can all be addressed with the use of a circular frame. Paley[64] reported 20 minor and major complications in 18 feet, with 25 various foot deformities treated with the Ilizarov apparatus. Patients must understand that the final functional outcome will be a stiff but cosmetically improved plantigrade foot. This treatment method is addressed in a separate article.

TRIPLE ARTHRODESIS

Triple arthrodesis, once the most commonly performed salvage procedure for resistant rigid clubfoot, is only considered when all other options have failed. This shift is because of reports of inevitable degenerative changes in the ankle and midfoot joints at long-term follow-up of these patients.[65] Rigid equinovarus deformity has been the most difficult deformity to correct with a triple arthrodesis, with 56% of patients having residual deformity after successful fusion. In the presence of symptomatic degeneration, a fusion becomes necessary and is effective at relieving pain. Associated procedures are used as required for optimum correction of the associated deformities.

SUMMARY

Based on the most recent information, initial soft tissue correction followed by extra-articular corrective osteotomies augmented by tendon rebalancing is the preferred treatment for achieving a plantigrade foot. Experts believe that for most patients, some motion from a stiff joint is better than no motion from a fused one. In the presence of symptomatic degeneration, however, a fusion is inevitable and will provide secure results when specific joints are fused in combination with other corrective procedures as required.

REFERENCES

1. Morcuende JA, Dolan LA, Dietz FR, et al. Radical reduction in the rate of extensive corrective surgery for clubfoot using the Ponseti method. Pediatrics 2004; 113:376–80.
2. Docquier PL, Leemrijse T, Rombouts JJ. Clinical and radiographic features of operatively treated stiff clubfeet after skeletal maturity: etiology of the deformities and how to prevent them. Foot Ankle Int 2006;27(1):29–37.
3. Ippolito E, Farsetti P, Caterini R, et al. Long-term comparative results in patients with congenital clubfoot treated with two different protocols. J Bone Joint Surg Am 2003;85:1286–94.
4. Swann M, Lloyd-Roberts GC, Catterall A. The anatomy of uncorrected club feet. A study of rotation deformity. J Bone Joint Surg Br 1969;51(2):263–9.
5. Pirani S, Zeznik L, Hodges D. Magnetic resonance imaging study of the congenital clubfoot treated with the Ponseti method. J Pediatr Orthop 2001;21:719–26.
6. Ponseti IV, El-Khoury GY, Ippolito E, et al. A radiographic study of skeletal deformities in treated clubfeet. Clin Orthop 1981;160:30–42.
7. Cummings RJ, Bashore CJ, Bookout CB, et al. Avascular necrosis of the talus after McKay clubfoot release for idiopathic congenital clubfoot. J Pediatr Orthop 2001;21(2):221–4.
8. Greider TD, Siff SJ, Gerson P, et al. Arteriography in club foot. J Bone Joint Surg Am 1982;64:837–40.

9. Aplington JP, Riddle CD Jr. Avascular necrosis of the body of the talus after combined medial and lateral release of congenital clubfoot. South Med J 1976; 69(8):1037–8.

10. Uglow MG, Clarke NM. The functional outcome of staged surgery for the correction of talipes equinovarus. J Pediatr Orthop 2000;20(4):517–23.

11. Kuo KN, Smith PA. Correcting residual deformity following clubfoot releases. Clin Orthop Relat Res 2009;467(5):1326–33.

12. El-Hawary R, Karol LA, Jeans KA, et al. Gait analysis of children treated for clubfoot with physical therapy or the Ponseti cast technique. J Bone Joint Surg Am 2008;90(7):1508–16.

13. Scher DM, Feldman DS, van Bosse HJ, et al. Predicting the need for tenotomy in the Ponseti method for correction of clubfeet. J Pediatr Orthop 2004;24(4): 349–52.

14. Goriainov V, Judd J, Uglow M. The value of initial Pirani Score Assessment of Clubfoot in predicting recurrence. Presented at British Society for Children's Orthopaedic Surgery. Birmingham (UK), January 23, 2009. Abstract to appear in Proceedings of JBJS Br.

15. Diméglio A, Bensahel H, Souchet P, et al. Classification of clubfoot. J Pediatr Orthop B 1995;4(2):129–36.

16. Dyer PJ, Davis N. The role of the Pirani scoring system in the management of club foot by the Ponseti method. J Bone Joint Surg Br 2006;88(8):1082–4.

17. Alvarez CM, De Vera MA, Chhina H, et al. The use of botulinum type A toxin in the treatment of idiopathic clubfoot: 5-year follow-up. J Pediatr Orthop 2009;29(6): 570–5.

18. Higginson JS, Zajac FE, Neptune RR, et al. Effect of equinus foot placement and intrinsic muscle response on knee extension during stance. Gait Posture 2006; 23(1):32–6.

19. Simbak N, Razak M. Residual deformity following surgical treatment of congenital talipes equinovarus. Med J Malaysia 1998;53(Suppl A):115–20.

20. Walling AK. The adult clubfoot (congenital pes cavus). Foot Ankle Clin 2008; 13(2):307–14, vii.

21. Mosca VS. The cavus foot. J Pediatr Orthop 2001;21(4):423–4.

22. Thompson GH, Hoyen HA, Barthel T. Tibialis anterior tendon transfer after clubfoot surgery. Clin Orthop Relat Res 2009;467(5):1306–13.

23. Wallander H, Aurell Y, Hansson G. No association between residual forefoot adduction and the position of the navicular in clubfeet treated by posterior release. J Pediatr Orthop 2007;27(1):60–6.

24. Otremski I, Salama R, Khermosh O, et al. Residual adduction of the forefoot. A review of the Turco procedure for congenital club foot. J Bone Joint Surg Br 1987;69(5):832–4.

25. Howlett JP, Mosca VS, Bjornson K. The association between idiopathic clubfoot and increased internal hip rotation. Clin Orthop Relat Res 2009;467(5):1231–7.

26. Sankar WN, Rethlefsen SA, Weiss J, et al. The recurrent clubfoot: can gait analysis help us make better preoperative decisions? Clin Orthop Relat Res 2009; 467(5):1214–22.

27. Haslam PG, Goddard M, Flowers MJ, et al. Overcorrection and generalized joint laxity in surgically treated congenital talipes equino-varus. J Pediatr Orthop B 2006;15(4):273–7.

28. El-Deeb KH, Ghoneim AS, El-Adwar KL, et al. Is it hazardous or mandatory to release the talocalcaneal interosseous ligament in clubfoot surgery: a preliminary report. J Pediatr Orthop 2007;27(5):517–21.

29. Kuo KN, Jansen LD. Rotatory dorsal subluxation of the navicular: a complication of clubfoot surgery. J Pediatr Orthop 1998;18(6):770–4.
30. McKay DW. Dorsal bunions in children. J Bone Joint Surg Am 1983;65(7):975–80.
31. Yong SM, Smith PA, Kuo KN. Dorsal bunion after clubfoot surgery: outcome of reverse Jones procedure. J Pediatr Orthop 2007;27(7):814–20.
32. Staheli LT, Corbett M, Wyss C, et al. Lower-extremity rotational problems in children. Normal values to guide management. J Bone Joint Surg Am 1985;67(1): 39–47.
33. Laaveg SJ, Ponseti IV. Long-term results of treatment of congenital club foot. J Bone Joint Surg Am 1980;62(1):23–31.
34. Cummings RJ, Davidson RS, Armstrong PF, et al. Congenital clubfoot. J Bone Joint Surg Am 2002;84(2):290–308.
35. Saltzman CL, el-Khoury GY. The hindfoot alignment view. Foot Ankle Int 1995; 16(9):572–6.
36. Ippolito E, Fraracci L, Farsetti P, et al. The influence of treatment on the pathology of club foot. CT study at maturity. J Bone Joint Surg Br 2004;86(4):574–80.
37. Sinclair MF, Bosch K, Rosenbaum D, et al. Pedobarographic analysis following Ponseti treatment for congenital clubfoot. Clin Orthop Relat Res 2009;467(5): 1223–30.
38. Dananberg HJ, Shearstone J, Guillano M. Manipulation method for the treatment of ankle equinus. J Am Podiatr Med Assoc 2000;90(8):385–9.
39. Spiegel DA, Shrestha OP, Sitoula P, et al. Ponseti method for untreated idiopathic clubfeet in Nepalese patients from 1 to 6 years of age. Clin Orthop Relat Res 2009;467(5):1164–70.
40. Karol LA, Concha MC, Johnston CE II. Gait analysis and muscle strength in children with surgically treated clubfeet. J Pediatr Orthop 1997;17(6):790–5.
41. Ferreira RC, Costa MT, Frizzo GG, et al. Correction of severe recurrent clubfoot using a simplified setting of the Ilizarov device. Foot Ankle Int 2007; 28(5):557–68.
42. Kumar PN, Laing PW, Klenerman L. Medial calcaneal osteotomy for relapsed equinovarus deformity. Long-term study of the results of Frederick Dwyer. J Bone Joint Surg Br 1993;75(6):967–71.
43. Dwyer FC. Osteotomy of the calcaneum for pes cavus. J Bone Joint Surg Br 1959;41:80–6.
44. El-Mowafi H. Assessment of percutaneous V osteotomy of the calcaneus with Ilizarov application for correction of complex foot deformities. Acta Orthop Belg 2004;70(6):586–90.
45. Kirienko A, Villa A, Calhoun JH. Ilizarov technique for complex foot and ankle deformities. New York (NY): Marcel Dekker, Inc; 2004.
46. Sherman FC, Westin GW. Plantar release in the correction of deformities of the foot in childhood. J Bone Joint Surg Am 1981;63(9):1382–9.
47. Fowler SB. The cavo-varus foot. J Bone Joint Surg Am 1959;41:757.
48. Barouk LS, Rippstein P, Toullec E. New proximal oblique metatarsal osteotomy for the treatment of pes cavus (brt osteotomy). J Bone Joint Surg Br 2002; 84B(Suppl 1):32–3.
49. Japas LM. Surgical treatment of pes cavus by tarsal V-osteotomy. Preliminary report. J Bone Joint Surg Am 1968;50(5):927–44.
50. Wilcox PG, Weiner DS. The Akron midtarsal dome osteotomy in the treatment of rigid pes cavus: a preliminary review. J Pediatr Orthop 1985;5(3):333–8.
51. Paley D, Tetsworth K. Percutaneous osteotomies. Osteotome and Gigli saw techniques. Orthop Clin North Am 1991;22:613–24.

52. Lu H, Qin L, Lee K, et al. Healing compared between bone to tendon and cartilage to tendon in a partial inferior patellectomy model in rabbits. Clin J Sport Med 2008;18(1):62–9.

53. Wicart PR, Barthes X, Ghanem I, et al. Clubfoot posteromedial release: advantages of tibialis anterior tendon lengthening. J Pediatr Orthop 2002;22(4):526–32.

54. Garceau CJ. Anterior tibial tendon transposition in recurrent congenital clubfoot. J Bone Joint Surg Am 1940;22:932–6.

55. Napiontek M, Kotwicki T, Tomaszewski M. Opening wedge osteotomy of the medial cuneiform before age 4 years in the treatment of forefoot adduction. J Pediatr Orthop 2003;23(1):65–9.

56. Mahadev A, Munajat I, Mansor A, et al. Combined lateral and transcuneiform without medial osteotomy for residual clubfoot for children. Clin Orthop Relat Res 2009;467(5):1319–25.

57. Lourenco AF, Dias LS, Zoellick DM, et al. Treatment of residual adduction deformity in clubfoot: the double osteotomy. J Pediatr Orthop 2001;21(6):713–8.

58. Evans D. Relapsed club foot. J Bone Joint Surg Br 1961;43:722–33.

59. Lichtblau S. A medial and lateral release operation for club foot: a preliminary report. J Bone Joint Surg Am 1973;55:1377–84.

60. Harvey AR, Uglow MG, Clarke NM. Clinical and functional outcome of relapse surgery in severe congenital talipes equinovarus. J Pediatr Orthop B 2003;12(1):49–55.

61. Mosca VS. Calcaneal lengthening for valgus deformity of the hind-foot. J Bone Joint Surg Am 1995;77:500–12.

62. Burghardt RD, Herzenberg JE, Standard SC, et al. Temporary hemiepiphyseal arrest using a screw and plate device to treat knee and ankle deformities in children: a preliminary report. J Child Orthop 2008;2(3):187–97.

63. Swaroop VT, Wenger DR, Mubarak SJ. Talonavicular fusion for dorsal subluxation of the navicular in resistant clubfoot. Clin Orthop Relat Res 2009;467(5):1314–8.

64. Paley D. The correction of complex foot deformities using Ilizarov's distraction osteotomies. Clin Orthop Relat Res 1993;293:97–111.

65. Saltzman CL, Fehrle MJ, Cooper RR, et al. Triple arthrodesis: twenty-five and forty-four-year average follow-up of the same patients. J Bone Joint Surg Am 1999;81(10):1391–402.

Ilizarov External Fixation in the Correction of Severe Pediatric Foot and Ankle Deformities

Sunil Dhar, MBBS, MS, MCh Orth, FRCS, FRCS Ed Orth

KEYWORDS

- Ilizarov • Foot and ankle • Deformity • Taylor spatial frame
- Pediatric • External fixation

The correction of complex foot and ankle deformities in children continues to be a difficult surgical challenge. A complex deformity is a multiplanar deformity with or without foot shortening.[1] A multiplanar foot deformity is defined by the presence of more than one deformity affecting the foot[2] (**Fig. 1**). These deformities may develop in any plane, including the coronal, sagittal, or transverse plane. Such deformities can be caused either primarily or be a sequel to congenital musculoskeletal conditions; neuromuscular disease; congenital talipes equinovarus (CTEV); trauma; infection, including osteomyelitis; and burn contractures. These deformities include deformed feet with poor soft-tissue coverage; relapsed or neglected cases; and those with accompanying problems, such as leg-length discrepancy, lower leg (supra malleolar) deformity, and nonunions.[3]

COMMON CONDITIONS

One of the most common causes of severe deformity of the foot and ankle in the pediatric population, until recently, has been the relapsed or neglected CTEV. With the current popularity worldwide of the Ponseti method of treatment of primary idiopathic CTEV, it is likely that the number of relapsed and severely deformed feet will diminish considerably. However, there sadly will remain large parts of our planet where such treatment is either unavailable or simply not socially acceptable or possible (compliance) and, therefore, one is likely to continue to be faced with such challenging cases.

The treatment of recurrent clubfoot is a challenge, even for experienced surgeons. This deformity has a tendency to recur even after several surgical attempts and often

Department of Trauma and Orthopaedics, Nottingham University Hospitals, Queen's Medical Centre Campus, Nottingham, NG7 2UH, UK
E-mail address: sunil.dhar@btinternet.com

Foot Ankle Clin N Am 15 (2010) 265–285
doi:10.1016/j.fcl.2010.03.001

foot.theclinics.com

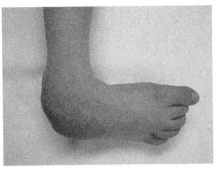

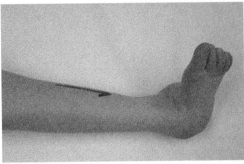

Fig. 1. A 5-year-old child with arthrogryposis. Severe, complex deformity of the right foot.

leads to a small, stiff, deformed foot. The complex, three-dimensional aspects of club-foot deformity allied to severe joint stiffness with contractures of the soft tissues, particularly in the multiply operated foot, significantly limits the use of conventional surgical corrective methods. Beware of aggressive correction of deformities by open surgical means because there is a considerable risk for damage to neurovascu-lar structures, which are usually embedded in scar tissue (**Fig. 2**). Excision of large bony wedges to correct deformity leads to further shortening of an already small foot. A significant limitation to the use of tarsal and metatarsal osteotomies and conventional arthrodesis to treat recurrent clubfoot is the considerable technical complexity, secondary to the three-dimensional aspects of the deformity. Potential risks to the soft tissues include extensive skin necrosis, secondary infection, neuro-vascular compromise, and ischemia, any of which may lead to amputation.[4–7]

Any paralytic or spastic disorder can lead to muscle imbalance and deformity of the foot and ankle (**Fig. 3**). Initially this may be a flexible deformity, but with skeletal growth bony deformities may occur secondary to soft-tissue and joint contractures leading to a stiff, deformed foot. If untreated, callus or skin ulceration, stress fractures of the metatarsals, joint instability, and other associated problems may develop. Patients may complain of pain, difficulty with shoe wear, decreased mobility, instability, gait abnormalities, and a poor cosmetic appearance.[2,8,9]

Neuromuscular conditions giving rise to foot and ankle deformities are numerous and these may be progressive or static in their manifestation. Common progressive conditions include the hereditary motor sensory neuropathies, such as Charcot-Marie-Tooth disease; myelomeningocele; syringomyelia; tethered cord; diastemato-myelia; and muscular dystrophy. The progressive nature of these disorders may affect the end results with some deterioration over time and thus patients have to be made

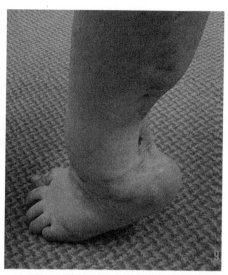

Fig. 2. A 15-year-old boy who suffered vascular compromise following repeat surgery for CTEV. He now has a single vessel foot with severe deformity, swelling and soft-tissue loss.

aware of this possibility. Common static causes include cerebral palsy; poliomyelitis; stroke; spinal cord or peripheral nerve injury; compartment syndrome; or iatrogenic causes (injection injury of the sciatic nerve).[8–11]

Surgical management is necessary for patients who have a deformity that causes functional disability. In the treatment of neuromuscular foot deformities, the goal is to provide a painless, plantigrade, stable foot that can fit into a shoe without undue difficulty. In general, the correction of neuromuscular foot deformities has involved soft-tissue releases, tendon transfers, osteotomies, or arthrodesis. However, in previously operated or severely rigid neuromuscular foot deformities, the soft tissues are contracted and there maybe bony deformity and joint involvement. In most of these patients, an appropriate correction cannot be obtained with soft-tissue procedures

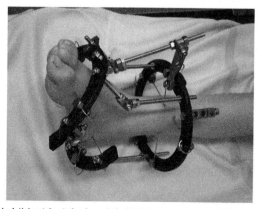

Fig. 3. A 9-year-old child with right hemiplegia and cavovarus deformity of the right foot. Undergoing correction in an Ilizarov frame.

alone and osteotomies or fusions are usually required. These methods, however, also reduce the size of the foot, frequently increasing the stiffness of the ankle and foot. Full correction of moderate to severe deformities is often difficult to obtain and complications, such as nonunion, residual deformity, recurrent deformity, ankle arthritis, and avascular necrosis of the talus, have been reported.[2,8–11]

There are several other conditions giving rise to significant and complex foot and ankle deformities in children. These include severe trauma[12]; burns with secondary contractures[13,14]; congenital conditions, such as fibular hemimelia[15] and sequel of severe infections (meningococcal and so forth); and osteomyelitis.[16] The basic principles of managing these deformities are essentially the same as outlined for the more common conditions.

COMPENSATORY MECHANISMS

Following deformity in one or more areas of the lower limb, compensatory adjustments in adjacent joints is a common phenomenon. Thus, a sagittal plane distal tibial deformity (eg, recurvatum) is usually compensated by ankle plantar flexion and distal tibial procurvatum by ankle dorsiflexion. A coronal plane distal tibial deformity (varus) often results in subtalar eversion and valgus in subtalar inversion to result in a plantigrade foot. Ankle equinus is often compensated by proximal (knee recurvatum, hip flexion and external rotation, exaggerated lordosis) or distal (midtarsal dorsiflexion) mechanisms. Cavus, driven either distally in the foot or proximally, can be compensated by a calcaneus or plantaris deformity, respectively. Hindfoot varus is compensated by forefoot pronation (cavovarus) and hindfoot valgus by forefoot supination (planovalgus). Conversely, forefoot pronation results in hindfoot varus and forefoot supination in hindfoot valgus. It is thus essential to assess for these compensations and the flexibility of joints, in particular the relationship of the forefoot to the hindfoot and if the deformities are flexible or fixed.[1,2,15]

CLASSIFICATION

Classification systems exist for developing treatment strategies for these complex deformities. Catagni and colleagues[17] divide foot and ankle deformity into five main types. They tailor their frame constructs accordingly.

Type 1 deformity: There is an alteration of the relationship of the foot to the tibia (eg, equinus deformity).
Type 2 deformity: There is a deformity within the foot without alteration of the relationship of the foot to the tibia (eg, cavus foot).
Type 3 deformity: There is deformity within the foot and an alteration of the relationship of the foot to the tibia (eg, fibular hemimelia, CTEV).
Type 4 deformity: There is a foot deformity secondary to a supramalleolar deformity and a supramalleolar osteotomy is required (eg, post pilon fracture).
Type 5 deformity: There is bone loss or absence within the foot and a reconstructive procedure is required (eg, post landmine blast injuries, calcaneal destruction, or congenital agenesis of the forefoot).

Beaman and Gellman[18] conceptualize foot and ankle deformity as a single-plane or a segmental deformity. The deformity may be bony or articular. A single-plane deformity is one where the foot can be corrected with one ring proximal and one ring distal to the level of deformity, for example, hindfoot varus as a result of a calcaneal malunion or an equinus (or equinovarus) deformity. A segmental deformity is one where there are two or more levels of deformity present each requiring a separate fixator construct to correct, for example, a triple arthrodesis malunion with asymmetric deformity between the hindfoot and forefoot or a clubfoot deformity with equinovarus and forefoot adduction. This method of conceptualization is helpful with preoperative planning of ring external fixator constructs.

THE METHOD OF ILIZAROV

Over the last 15 years or so, gradual correction of complex foot and ankle deformities, using the principles of Ilizarov, has transformed our ability to deal with these difficult clinical problems.[15,16] The discovery of distraction histogenesis and the development of the circular fine-wire external fixator has allowed for correction of complex deformities of the foot and ankle, including the ability to perform gradual correction and to modify treatment during correction while allowing early weight bearing once correction is achieved.[19,20] Foot length can be maintained or gained. During the course of correction, a gradual lengthening of the soft tissues, including blood vessels, nerves, muscles, connective tissues, and skin occurs, reducing the risks for neurovascular damage, skin necrosis, and secondary infection. The Ilizarov method is safe and minimally invasive, requiring minimal or no bone resection resulting in more predictable and satisfactory results at least in the medium term.[15,16,19,20]

Correction of foot and ankle deformity with circular frames in children should not be considered a one off treatment but part of an ongoing management plan that requires regular assessment until skeletal maturity, ongoing orthotic support, and occasionally further surgery. The latter should not necessarily be considered a failure of the ring fixator treatment.

TREATMENT STRATEGIES AND PRINCIPLES

The aim of treatment is to achieve a plantigrade, stable foot that is painless and allows patients to achieve good function. Treatment strategies essentially depend on four factors: the age of the child, the severity of the deformity, the stiffness of the joints of the foot and ankle, and the etiology of the condition.

There are two approaches to correct deformities of the foot in children with the Ilizarov apparatus: with or without osteotomy.[21] In the non-osteotomy method the deformity is corrected by distracting the foot joints and their soft tissues, thus avoiding compressive forces across the joints. Differential distraction of soft tissues is a powerful technique to achieve correction; for example, more rapid distraction on the concave side of the deformity than the convex side in a bean-shaped foot eventually results in deformity correction. This technique is thus applicable in younger patients (under 10 years of age) with mainly soft-tissue and joint contractures, rather than major bone deformities. In these patients there remains the potential to remodel bone deformity and achieve joint congruity, which is thought to occur by activation of the circumferential physis of these bones.[21] In the osteotomy distraction technique, the deformity is corrected through the osteotomy. Osteotomy distraction is preferred in cases with bone deformity in children (usually more than 10 years of age); in patients with neuromuscular imbalance in whom tendon transfers alone would not maintain correction; in severely stiff feet; and in cases with previous fusions or nonunions.

Four basic distraction foot osteotomy levels have been described for correction of foot deformities[1]: supramalleolar,[2] hindfoot,[3] forefoot (midfoot),[4] and combined hind and forefoot (midfoot) (**Fig. 4**). Supramalleolar osteotomies are indicated when there is a supramalleolar deformity and can also be used for derotation and limb lengthening. Hindfoot osteotomies include the calcaneal osteotomy, the U-shaped

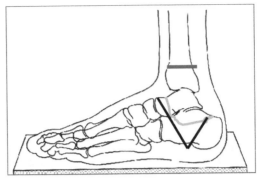

Fig. 4. Osteotomy types: red indicate supramalleolar, green indicates U-shaped osteotomy, blue indicates V-shaped osteotomy.

osteotomy and the V-shaped osteotomy. The U-shaped osteotomy (**Fig. 5**) passes under the subtalar joint through the superior part of the calcaneum and across the sinus tarsi out through the neck of the talus. It is indicated when there is associated talar deformity, such as a flat top talus, and therefore limited scope for ankle movement. The deformities are corrected through the U-shaped osteotomy, leaving the ankle in its original position. The V-shaped osteotomy (**Fig. 6**) is a double osteotomy, proximally across the body of the calcaneum and distally across the neck of the talus

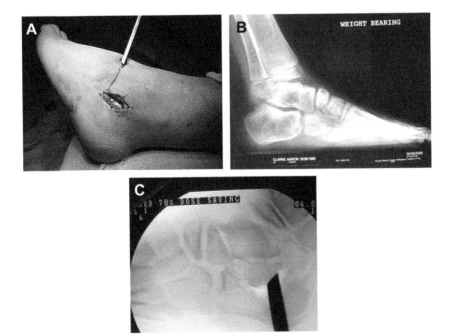

Fig. 5. A 12-year-old child post several operations for CTEV (*A*). Complex deformity with hindfoot varus and equinus. Note that there is no potential to correct equinus at the ankle (*B*). The subtalar joint is nonfunctional and stiff. A U-shaped osteotomy can be used to correct the deformities (*C*).

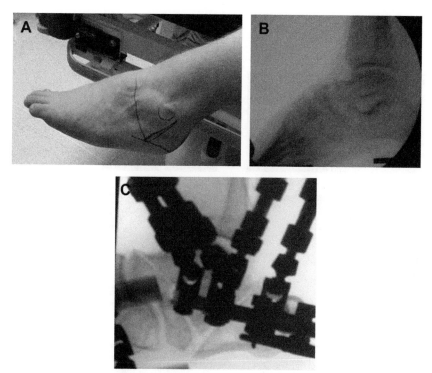

Fig. 6. 15-year-old child post operation with residual deformities from CTEV (*A*). Note severe hindfoot varus, plantaris, and supination deformities (*B*). A V-shaped osteotomy is ideal for correction of these deformities with little compromise of the midfoot joints (*C*).

or the midfoot. The two converge on the plantar aspect of the calcaneum. It is indicated when there are hindfoot and forefoot deformities.[15,21] Both the U-shaped and the V-shaped osteotomies cross the subtalar joint and hence potentially stiffen it and should, therefore, only be performed if the subtalar joint is stiff or fused to begin with. However, most subtalar joints in severe deformities are stiff or ankylosed anyway. We prefer the V-shaped osteotomy to the U-shaped osteotomy because it is much easier to control. In addition, in our experience the incidence of premature consolidation is high with the U-shaped osteotomy because it can be quite a challenge to get it to move along its arc and the frame configuration can get complicated.

In performing an osteotomy, it is important to minimize thermal necrosis and periosteal damage by avoiding the use of power saws. The multiple drill hole and osteotome technique is commonly used in the calcaneum and the neck of the talus. The Gigli saw technique (**Fig. 7**) is useful in the midfoot because ensuring completeness of the osteotomy using an osteotome is quite difficult and one of the reasons for premature consolidation of the osteotomy.[22] The osteotomy usually is performed from medial to lateral but may be done from lateral to medial. Four incisions are made: dorsomedial, dorsolateral, plantar medial, and plantar lateral. The flexible Gigli saw is passed dorsally via the dorsolateral incision, delivered via the dorsomedial incision, then out via the plantar medial incision, and finally back out through the plantar lateral incision all the while carefully staying as close to bone as possible to minimize the potential for neurovascular injury. This technique may be used in the region between the talar neck and the tarsometatarsal joints.

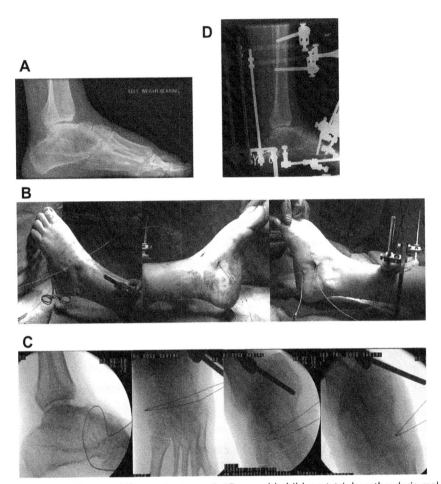

Fig. 7. The Gigli saw midfoot osteotomy. A 15-year-old child post triple arthrodesis mal-union (*A*). A midfoot osteotomy was performed to correct a supination and plantaris defor-mity. Gigli saw introduced from lateral to medial on the dorsal surface, delivered through a plantar medial portals, and then passed back to the lateral side on the plantar surface (*B*). Preoperative radiographs show the progression of the osteotomy (*C*). Completed osteot-omy (*D*).

PREOPERATIVE ASSESSMENT

A thorough history and examination often establishes the cause of deformity. Differing pathologies respond differently during the deformity-correction process, often with the congenital ones being the most challenging. The patients' main complaint is iden-tified together with their expectations from treatment so that an objective can be established for any proposed surgery. Clinical examination should evaluate the components of any deformity; forefoot-hindfoot relationships (eg, the Coleman block test); ankle, subtalar, midtarsal and toe joints ranges of movement; the level of any equinus deformity; and the condition of the skin and soft tissues. A complete radio-graphic evaluation is important. Weight-bearing ankle and foot radiographs including a hindfoot alignment view are essential. The hindfoot alignment view (**Fig. 8**) is useful

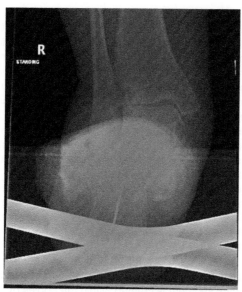

Fig. 8. The hindfoot alignment view. The relationship between the long axis of the calcaneum and tibia along with any ankle (and subtalar joint, by inference) deformity can be readily assessed.

to evaluate tibia, ankle, and calcaneal deformity.[23] A line on the vertical axis of the midbody of the calcaneus should be parallel and approximately 1 cm lateral to the middiaphyseal line of the tibia. Valgus deformity and lateral translation occur with a pes planus deformity; varus angulation and medial translation occur with a cavovarus type deformity.[18] In severe deformities, radiographs are often difficult to interpret and a CT reconstruction may be helpful. Although an MRI is not routine on our unit, it may be helpful if infection, tumor, and cartilage pathology are suspected.

OPERATIVE TECHNIQUE

There are essentially two circular frame types currently used in clinical practice: the standard Ilizarov frame and the recently developed Taylor Spatial Frame (TSF) (Smith & Nephew, Memphis, TN, USA). The Ilizarov frame has been used for more than 50 years; however, the TSF is a relative newcomer with less than 10 years in foot and ankle practice. Both methods are valid techniques and appropriate for treating what can be challenging deformities. Both require meticulous preoperative planning for the relevant osteotomies and accurate placement of wires and rings. The Ilizarov technique is more intuitive and surgeon dependent to determine hinge placement and the rate of distraction. The TSF is a computer-program driven circular frame that corrects deformities around a virtual hinge. The choice of which frame to use is a matter of personal preference and experience.

Ilizarov Frame

Our standard frame is constructed preoperatively and follows the following principles: rings mimic the deformities (orthogonal to respective segments); fixation adjacent to osteotomies to prevent joint subluxation; hydroxyapatite (HA)-coated half pins (improved pull out strength, reduced pin-site infection); motors and hinges to provide mainly differential distraction; and building the frame anticipating any potential future modifications (**Fig. 9**). Ilizarov frames can be of two types: a constrained frame or an unconstrained frame. In a constrained frame, mainly single-axis hinges are used and the deformity is corrected around the hinge axes, such as when an osteotomy is performed or in neuromuscular feet. In contrast, the joints of the foot and ankle serve as the hinge in an unconstrained design. An unconstrained frame is useful for soft-tissue distraction in children aged 10 years and younger and uses universal hinges that allow movement in all axes.

The frame consists of three main parts: a tibial base construct, a heel construct, and forefoot construct. We use a single ring for the tibial base in most children although two rings can be used in the bigger child. A single transverse olive wire and two HA-coated half pins are used to secure the tibial ring. The heel construct is a half ring or two-thirds ring attached to the calcaneum by two olive wires and an additional half pin along the long axis of the calcaneum, if required. The forefoot part of the frame usually consists of a half ring attached to two olive wires inserted transversely through the metatarsal shafts. In severely deformed feet, a full ring can be used to obtain a more stable construct. One wire is inserted through the first and fifth metatarsals distally, and one is placed as close as possible to the midfoot osteotomy. With U- or V-shaped osteotomy or a combination of midfoot and calcaneal osteotomies, a triangular middle bone segment is created within the bodies of the talus and calcaneus. This mobile bone segment should be stabilized with an olive wire or a half pin, and connected to the tibial base frame, to enable correction of the hindfoot and forefoot segments relative to the middle segment. Appropriate hinges and motors are attached between the three constructs to drive the deformity correction. It is essential that the posterior motors between the tibial and the hindfoot constructs be inclined

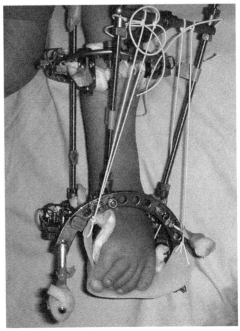

Fig. 9. Ilizarov external fixator correction of a severely deformed foot following an arterial embolic phenomenon caused by umbilical cord cannulisation.

posteriorly to prevent pushing the talus forward out of the ankle joint during correction. A full description of hinge and motor placement is clearly beyond the scope of this article (**Fig. 10**).

Taylor Spatial Frame

There are many possible frame configurations with the TSF in the correction of foot and ankle deformities (**Fig. 11**). The 6 + 6 configuration (**Fig. 12**) is commonly used, where the forefoot and the hindfoot are separately connected to the tibial base ring with no connection between them. It is useful for the gradual correction of soft-tissue deformities or to drive foot osteotomies, such as a V-type osteotomy of the hindfoot/midfoot. The miter frame configuration (**Fig. 13**) consists of two two-thirds rings over the foot and one full tibial ring. It allows correction of tibial alignment with the hindfoot correction (equinus and supramalleolar deformity) and hindfoot to forefoot alignment (cavus, forefoot adduction, supination). The butt frame configuration (**Fig. 14**) consists of a U plate over the foot connected to standard rings over the tibia and foot. This configuration allows correction of midfoot and forefoot deformities alone or in combination with correction more proximally (supramalleolar level). A special modification of the butt frame referred to as the "Tennessee Torpedo" (**Fig. 15**) is a versatile design for osteotomy corrections in the foot but is too bulky and heavy for use in children.[18] This frame configuration consists of two U rings connected at right angles, with one ring connected orthogonally to the distal tibia and the other, a stirrup ring, connected to the talus and calcaneus. From this base, a ring can be extended posteriorly to allow gradual correction of a calcaneal osteotomy and a ring can be attached to the forefoot for correction of any midfoot deformity. This fixator construct can be used with forefoot and hindfoot deformity corrections, as with a segmental deformity, or with only the hindfoot portion or the forefoot portion. The location of the stirrup or butt ring into the talus and calcaneus can be moved proximally or distally in the foot if only the hindfoot or forefoot portions are used. TSF struts and the online software program are used in the gradual correction of deformity with these frame configurations. After foot-deformity correction and achieving a plantigrade position, the frame is modified to place a standard foot ring to allow weight bearing and correction of any equinus deformity.

The Ponse-Taylor method of correction of foot deformity, introduced by Herzenberg in 2003, is an application of Ponseti principles using a TSF and consists of two

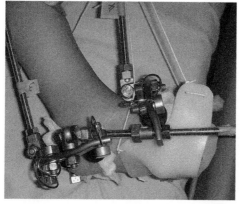

Fig. 10. Ilizarov motors and hinges to assist with deformity correction.

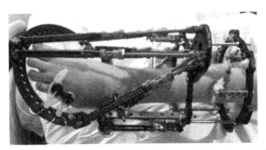

Fig. 11. Taylor Spatial Frame for correction of hindfoot and forefoot deformities. The talus has been stabilized with a half pin.

stages.[24,25] It includes initial correction of internal tibial torsion, hindfoot varus, distraction of subtalar joint, and partial correction of the equinus. During the first stage, a talar wire (olive wire inserted laterally) is attached to the proximal ring to allow derotation of the foot. At this stage, the equinus is corrected just to neutral. Before proceeding to the second stage, full correction of the rotation and varus should be achieved. In the second stage, the remaining equinus is corrected after frame modification (talar neck wire applied to the distal ring to allow hindfoot dorsiflexion).

POSTOPERATIVE CARE

Correction begins on the second postoperative day, and should proceed as rapidly as soft-tissue adaptation and patient tolerance allows. The majority of patients receive a popliteal nerve block at induction in theater for postoperative pain control. In the immediate postoperative period, morphine is used through patient-controlled analgesia (PCA), which is gradually substituted by oral analgesia (paracetamol, codeine-based). Patients and care givers are instructed about pin-site care and rate of distraction. Our pin-site protocol is to clean the sites of the wires and half pins using a normal saline solution and to apply a compressive dressing of chlorhexidine-soaked gauze once per week or more often if there is any evidence of discharge or pin-site infection. The correction is monitored at regular intervals with radiographs and observed for epiphysiolysis (commonly distal tibial), ankle, or midtarsal subluxation. Regular physiotherapy is commenced to prevent knee or toe contractures and patients are encouraged to mobilize weight bearing as tolerated once the foot is

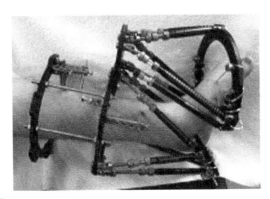

Fig. 12. 6 + 6 TSF.

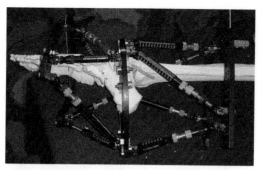

Fig. 13. Saw bone model of TSF miter frame.

plantigrade. Because of the tendency for tissues to recoil, overcorrection[5,26,27] of deformity is planned. After deformity correction, the static frame is maintained for 6 weeks followed by removal and short leg plaster for 6 weeks. To maintain the correction and avoid early recurrence, a rigid ankle foot orthosis is worn day and night for 6 to 12 months and then at night only for several years.[5,28,29]

COMPLICATIONS

Complications are frequent with Ilizarov fixation but most of them are minor and do not alter or affect the outcome of treatment. Intraoperative neurovascular injury can be avoided by following safe anatomic windows while inserting wires. Common problems encountered during the distraction phase are pin tract infections and toe contractures, occasionally complicated by metatarsophalangeal (MTP) subluxation.[3,5,28] Pin-tract problems are related to skin motion at the interface, often observed in the metatarsal wires.[30] Superficial pin-tract infections are managed with regular pin-site care and oral antibiotics. Systemic antibiotics are administered for deep infection that may need removal of the wire in resistant cases. Toe contractures are treated by passive stretching and toe slings. Persistent toe contractures are treated by flexor tendon release or

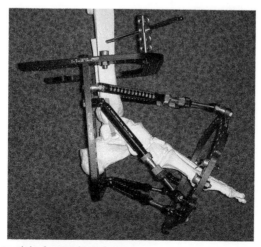

Fig. 14. Saw bone model of a TSF butt frame.

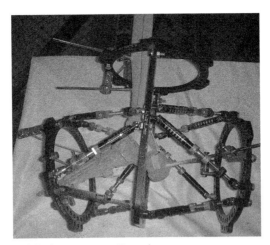

Fig. 15. Saw bone model of a Tennessee Torpedo.

lengthening.[29] Prophylactic k-wiring of the toes (**Fig. 16**) helps to reduce this complication. Metatarsophalangeal subluxation may require closed or open reduction and
pinning.[3,28] Hosny[30] persisted with aggressive physiotherapy and splintage and noted
MTP joint reduction after fixator removal.

Ankle subluxation, premature consolidation at the osteotomy site,[26,30,31] and epiphysiolysis[5,28,32] are rare but significant complications that should be watched out
for. Subluxation at ankle or midtarsal level requires acute reduction and readjustment
of the frame.[29] Epiphysiolysis is often noted in rigid deformities.[32] Choi and
colleagues[32] advocate a transepiphyseal wire to prevent it but there is a risk for septic
arthritis caused by pin-tract infection. Premature consolidation is avoided by making
certain that the osteotomy is complete initially, commencing distraction from day 2
post operation, ensuring the frame construct drives the osteotomy, and maintaining
a satisfactory distraction rate. The latter is patient and soft-tissue dependent, because
too rapid a rate often results in pain and may cause soft-tissue necrosis and further
scarring.

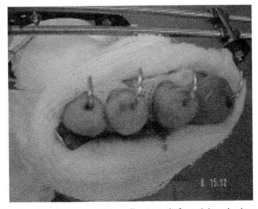

Fig. 16. Prophylactic pinning to prevent toe flexion deformities during frame correction.

Asymptomatic bone cysts have been observed in the lateral metatarsals, often in the base of the fifth metatarsal, following Ilizarov distraction for recurrent clubfoot deformities. The cysts appeared during or after treatment and had not resolved by the 3-year follow-up.[33,34] MRI[34] suggests the cysts were filled with fat, and histologic examination[33] revealed empty lacuna with no cell lining. Local vascular impairment[30] and disuse osteopenia theories[34] were proposed but the cause remains elusive.

LITERATURE REVIEW

There is no standardized evaluation available to assess the correction of neglected or recurrent clubfeet. Most studies have used subjective evaluation and so it is difficult to compare the results between various studies and techniques. However, the Ilizarov technique is often used as a salvage option where conventional techniques have failed and most of the literature reports successful correction, even in the most severe deformities. Several studies have reported satisfactory results of Ilizarov method for the treatment of resistant or neglected clubfeet (**Figs. 17** and **18**).

Franke and colleagues[35] reported the treatment outcome of 12 subjects with clubfeet who were aged 8 to 15 years. The authors used 4 to 10 weeks of distraction with an additional 8 to 10 weeks in a frame with the foot in a fixed position. Correction with a plantigrade foot and normal shoe wearing were achieved in all cases.

Bradish and Noor[5] reported excellent to good results in 75% of 17 relapsed clubfeet with Ilizarov method at 3 years. Split tibialis anterior tendon transfer was performed on five mobile feet that appeared to be effective in preventing the recurrence.

Choi and colleagues[32] reviewed the results of medial release and Ilizarov fixation on 12 recurrent arthrogrypotic clubfeet. Only one recurrence was reported up to 35 months. They have modified the fixation by transfixing the talus with olive wire and pulled medially to facilitate the derotation of talus. The mean American Orthopedic Foot and Ankle Society (AOFAS) foot score improved from 57 to 88 but stiffness at ankle and subtalar joint persisted.

Nakase and colleagues[36] reported a 360-degree release around the subtalar joint and Ilizarov fixation for recurrent clubfeet in older children (aged 4–10 years). All six feet except one achieved and maintained plantigrade position with more than twofold increase in ankle movement at 5-years follow-up.

Prem and colleagues[27] noted excellent to good results in 70% (14 out of 19) of recurrent clubfeet treated with soft tissue Ilizarov distraction. This study is the only one with long–term follow-up (5–10 years), and assessment was done using the international clubfoot study group score. Despite good results, reduced movement at ankle and subtalar joint were noted. They have associated limited ankle dorsiflexion with flat top talus that seems to be the effect rather than the cause of the problem.

Ferreira and colleagues[28] reported 77% good results of 35 recurrent clubfeet in older children (aged 14 years) at 56-months follow-up. In addition to plantar fasciotomy and Achilles tenotomy, 11 feet required midfoot osteotomy. However, recurrence was noted in one third and 13 feet required arthrodesis for symptomatic arthritis or recurrence.

Freedman and colleagues[37] reported 86% fair to poor outcome with Ilizarov method for resistant clubfoot at 6.6-years follow-up. This result may be related to a markedly reduced time in the frame (28 days) and no postoperative splintage.

Subjective and objective evaluation may not always correlate. Despite a 70% (12 out of 17) recurrence rate after soft-tissue distraction and 55% (5 out of 9) following bony distraction, patients' subjective satisfaction was reported as good by Utukuri and colleagues[29]

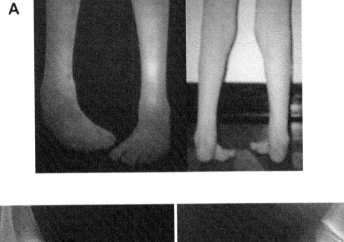

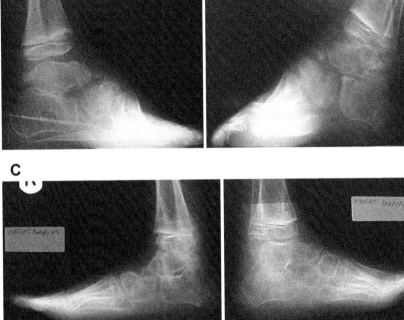

Fig. 17. A 7-year-old child with arthrogryposis and severe bilateral foot and ankle deformities (*A*). Preoperative lateral radiographs show widespread bony abnormalities following attempted surgeries at deformity correction (*B*). Post Ilizarov frame correction lateral radiographs show a plantigrade feet with subtalar ankylosis (*C*). Antero posterior radiographs of feet showing significant metatarsus adductus (*D*). Post Ilizarov correction showing a satisfactory result (*E*). Final pictures showing plantigrade feet (*F*).

In neuromuscular disorders, there is a high risk for recurrence following correction of the deformity caused by neuromuscular imbalance. Song and colleagues[38] reported on correction of severe equinovarus deformity with limb lengthening in 14 post poliomyelitis feet. More complications were observed with soft-tissue distraction (5 out of 7) compared with 85% (6 out of 7) good results with triple arthrodesis. The complications included equinus contracture, knee flexion contracture, and anterior subluxation of talus.

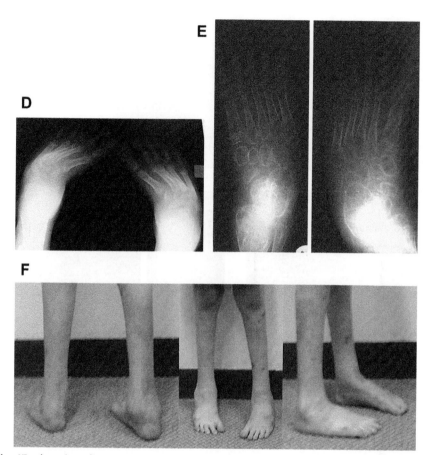

Fig. 17. (*continued*)

Biedermann and colleagues[39] noted a high recurrence rate of equinus (58%) in spastic diplegics and hemiplegics following initial good correction using Ilizarov soft-tissue distraction. This recurrence rate was much higher than other surgical methods. The deformity recurrence is attributed to abnormal muscle tone and bone growth in children. They recommended the Ilizarov technique be reserved for resistant cases.[33]

Burns contracture affecting the foot and ankle can lead to equinus, cavus, rocker bottom, toe dislocations, and limb length discrepancy. Equinus is common and caused by posterior scar contracture, anterior leg muscle loss, post burn positioning, or tibial growth in a rigid unyielding scar. The frame constitutes two tibial rings, one calcaneal half ring, and one metatarsal half ring with universal hinges and rods as described for clubfoot correction. Correction is achieved by anterior compression and posterior distraction. To avoid anterior tibiotalar compression and articular damage, the ankle requires 3 to 5 mm of distraction.[13,14] In addition, posteriorly inclined distraction prevents anterior subluxation of talus.[13,38,40] After correction of deformity, the frame is left in place for 6 weeks followed by a short leg cast for 6 weeks. Physical therapy and long-term orthotics are essential to prevent recurrence. Carmichael and

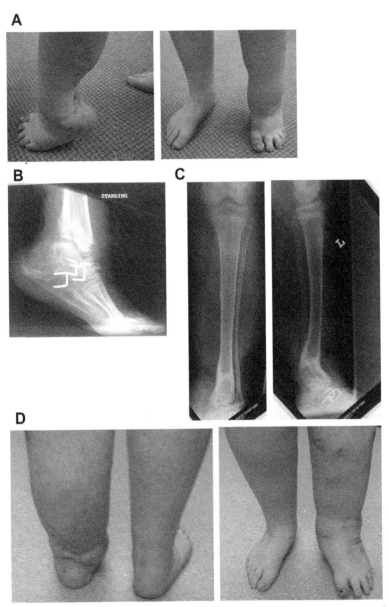

Fig. 18. 15-year-old boy with residual deformities following several operations on his left foot for CTEV, resulting in a vascular episode and severe soft-tissue and bony damage (*A*). Preoperative lateral radiograph (*B*). Given the overall clinical picture, the decision was made to give him a plantigrade foot via a supramalleolar osteotomy, gradually distracted in an Ilizarov frame. Final radiographs and clinical pictures (*C, D*).

colleagues[14] reported a 74% (17 out of 23) recurrence in pediatric patients at 46-months follow-up. The mean equinus improved from 34 degrees to 7 degrees of dorsiflexion but the deformity recurred quickly at a mean time of 17 months. The recurrence was caused by unyielding soft tissues and continued bone growth.

SUMMARY

Most of the evidence to date on the Ilizarov method in the management of complex foot and ankle deformities in children is based on expert opinion and retrospective case series. Often the technique is used as a salvage option where conventional techniques are inappropriate or have failed. The decision to use the Ilizarov external fixator to an alternative technique depends on several issues: complexity of the pathology, patient compliance, surgeon skills, and the capacity of the institution to manage patients with multidisciplinary requirements. Nevertheless, the Ilizarov method has proved to be a valuable tool for the satisfactory management of many previously unresolved clinical problems. With greater experience and further developments, the exact place of this powerful treatment modality will become clearer and even more successful.

REFERENCES

1. Shalaby H, Hefny H. Correction of complex foot deformities using the V-osteotomy and the Ilizarov technique. Strategies Trauma Limb Reconstr 2007;2:21–3.
2. Kucukkaya M, Kuzgun U. Neuromuscular deformity: treatment with external fixation. Foot Ankle Clin 2009;14(3):1447–70.
3. Kocaoglu M, Eralp L, Atalar AC, et al. Correction of complex foot deformities using the Ilizarov external fixator. J Foot Ankle Surg 2002;41:30–9.
4. Silver L, Grant AD, Atar D, et al. Use of tissue expansion in clubfoot surgery. Foot Ankle 1993;14:117–22.
5. Bradish CF, Noor S. The Ilizarov method in the management of relapsed club feet. J Bone Joint Surg Br 2000;82:387–91.
6. Uglow MG, Clarke NM. Relapse in staged surgery for congenital equinovarus. J Bone Joint Surg Br 2000;82:739–43.
7. Ilizarov GA, Shevtsov VI, Kuźmin NV. Method of treating talipes equinocavus. Ortop Travmatol Protez 1983;5:46–8.
8. Frawley PA, Broughton NS, Menelaus MB. Incidence and type of hindfoot deformities in patients with low-level spina bifida. J Pediatr Orthop 1998;18(3):312–3.
9. Horstmann HM. Neuromuscular foot deformities in children. In: Gould JS, Their SO, editors. Operative foot surgery. Philadelphia: WB Saunders; 1994. p. 797–833.
10. Beals TC, Nickisch F. Charcot-Marie-Tooth disease and the cavovarus foot. Foot Ankle Clin 2008;13(2):259–74.
11. Dehne R. Congenital and acquired neurologic disorders. In: Coughlin MJ, Their SO, editors. Surgery of the foot and ankle. 8th edition. Philadelphia: Mosby; 2007. p. 1761–806.
12. Beals TC. Applications of ring fixators in complex foot and ankle trauma. Orthop Clin North Am 2001;32:205–14.
13. Calhoun JH, Evans EB, Herndon DN. Techniques for the management of burn contractures with the Ilizarov fixator. Clin Orthop 1992;280:117–24.
14. Carmichael KD, Maxwell SC, Calhoun JH. Recurrence rates of burn contracture ankle equinus and other foot deformities in children treated with Ilizarov fixation. J Pediatr Orthop 2005;25:523–8.
15. Paley D. Principles of deformity correction. Berlin: Springer-Verlag; 2002.
16. Kirienko A, Villa A, Calhoun JH. Ilizarov technique for complex foot and ankle deformities. Philadelphia: Taylor & Francis, Inc; 2004. p. 2–6.
17. Catagni MA, Guerreschi F, Manzotti A, et al. Treatment of foot deformities using the Ilizarov method. Foot and Ankle Surgery 2000;6:207–37.

18. Beaman DN, Gellman R. The basics of ring external fixator application and care. Foot Ankle Clin 2008;13:15–27.
19. Ilizarov GA. The tension stress effect on the genesis and growth of tissues: part I – the influence of stability of fixation and soft tissue preservation. Clin Orthop 1989; 238:249.
20. Ilizarov GA. The tension stress effect on the genesis and growth of tissues: part II – the influence of the rate and frequency of distraction. Stability of fixation and soft tissue preservation. Clin Orthop 1989;239:263.
21. Paley D. The correction of complex foot deformities using Ilizarov's distraction osteotomies. Clin Orthop 1993;293:97–111.
22. Paley D, Herzenberg JE. Application of external fixation to foot and ankle reconstruction. In: Meyerson MS, Their SO, editors. Foot and ankle disorders. Philadelphia: WB Saunders; 2000. p. 1135–88.
23. Saltzman CL, El-Khoury GY. The hindfoot alignment view. Foot Ankle Int 1995;16: 572–6.
24. Eidelman M, Katzman A, Bor N, et al. Treatment of residual clubfoot deformities with the Taylor spatial frame using a Ponseti sequence. Poster presented at European Paediatric Orthopaedic Society 26th Annual Meeting. Sorrento, Italy, April 11–14, 2007.
25. Ponseti IV. Congenital clubfoot: fundamentals of treatment. New York: Oxford University Press; 1996.
26. Grant AD, Atar D, Lehman WB. The Ilizarov technique in correction of complex foot deformities. Clin Orthop 1992;280:94–116.
27. Prem H, Zenios M, Farrell R, et al. Soft tissue Ilizarov correction of congenital talipes equinovarus–5 to 10 years post-surgery. J Pediatr Orthop 2007;27: 220–4.
28. Ferreira RC, Costa MT, Frizzo GG, et al. Correction of severe recurrent clubfoot using a simplified setting of the Ilizarov device. Foot Ankle Int 2007;28: 557–68.
29. Utukuri MM, Ramachandran M, Hartley J, et al. Patient based outcomes after Ilizarov surgery in resistant clubfeet. J Pediatr Orthop B 2006;15:278–84.
30. Hosny GA. Correction of foot deformities by the Ilizarov method without corrective osteotomies or soft tissue release. J Pediatr Orthop B 2002;11:121–8.
31. O'Doherty DP, Street R, Saleh M. The use of circular external fixators in the management of complex disorders of the foot and ankle. The Foot 1992;2: 135–42.
32. Choi IH, Yang MS, Chung CY, et al. The treatment of recurrent arthrogrypotic clubfoot in children by the Ilizarov method. J Bone Joint Surg Br 2001;83: 731–7.
33. Ganel A, Grogan D, Guidera K, et al. Residual bone cysts after correction of severe foot deformities with the Ilizarov technique. J Pediatr Orthop 1997;17: 25–8.
34. Bradish CF, Tan S. Residual bone cysts after Ilizarov treatment of relapsed clubfeet. J Pediatr Orthop 2001;21:218–20.
35. Franke J, Grill F, Hein G, et al. Correction of clubfoot relapse using Ilizarov's apparatus in children 8-15 years old. Arch Orthop Trauma Surg 1990;110:33–7.
36. Nakase T, Yasui N, Ohzono K, et al. Treatment of relapsed idiopathic clubfoot by complete subtalar release combined with the Ilizarov method. J Foot Ankle Surg 2006;45:337–41.
37. Freedman JA, Watts H, Otsuka NY. The Ilizarov method for the treatment of resistant clubfoot: is it an effective solution? J Pediatr Orthop 2006;26:432–7.

38. Song HY, Myrboh V, Oh CW, et al. Tibial lengthening and concomitant foot deformity correction in 14 patients with permanent deformity after poliomyelitis. Acta Orthop 2005;76:261–9.
39. Biedermann R, Kaufmann G, Lair J, et al. High recurrence after calf lengthening with the Ilizarov apparatus for treatment of spastic equinus foot deformity. J Pediatr Orthop B 2007;16:125–8.
40. Laughlin RT, Calhoun JH. Ring fixators for reconstruction of traumatic disorders of the foot and ankle. Orthop Clin North Am 1995;26:287–94.

The Adult Sequelae of Treated Congenital Clubfoot

James W. Brodsky, MD[a,b],*

KEYWORDS

• Talipes equinovarus • Clubfoot • Arthritis • Arthrodesis

A great deal is known about the presentation, pathophysiologic variations, and treatments of congenital idiopathic clubfoot. Although much less ample, there are reports, as well as series, of these cases followed over intermediate and long-term intervals.[1] These reports indicate satisfactory functional results but with a high rate both of residual deformities, especially hindfoot varus, and of residual radiographic abnormalities, particularly deformation of the talar dome.[1–4]

Much less is known about the nature of the problems in these patients when functional results deteriorate or are unsatisfactory later in life. There are limited studies about the incidence, nature, and severity of symptoms in adults with treated clubfoot; the rate at which symptoms increase and function diminishes with advancing age; and the appropriate treatments.

It is easier to pose most of these questions of incidence than answer them. However, a retrospective examination of similar cases that have been presented for treatment may advance the goal of describing the nature of some of the late-appearing problems experienced by adults who were treated in childhood for congenital idiopathic talipes equinovarus.

There has been far more written on the treatment of untreated congenital talipes equinovarus in adults than on the treatment of adults who had treatment as a child and then developed subsequent problems in adolescence or adulthood.[5–7] The same is true about acquired or developmental adult cavovarus deformities of neurologic or traumatic origin.[6,8]

In the previously untreated clubfoot of a skeletally mature individual, the issue is one of achieving correction of a complex combination of deformities, including equinus, varus, and cavus. This almost invariably requires combinations of bony and soft tissue

[a] Foot and Ankle Surgery Fellowship Program, Baylor University Medical Center, 3900 Junius Street, #500, 411 North Washington Avenue, Suite 2100, Dallas, TX 75246, USA
[b] Department of Orthopaedic Surgery, University of Texas Southwestern Medical School, 3900 Junius Street #500, Dallas, TX 75246, USA
* Foot and Ankle Surgery Fellowship Program, Baylor University Medical Center, 3900 Junius Street, #500, 411 North Washington Avenue, Suite 2100, Dallas, TX 75246.
E-mail address: footandanklefellowship@gmail.com

Foot Ankle Clin N Am 15 (2010) 287–296
doi:10.1016/j.fcl.2010.03.002
1083-7515/10/$ – see front matter © 2010 Published by Elsevier Inc.

foot.theclinics.com

deformities, as well as considerations of tendon transfer, to address the frequently occurring neurologic component of the deformity. In years past, these cases have been seen frequently in the southwestern states of United States because of their proximity to immigrant Latin American populations. In many ways, these cases are more easily identified and their treatment more easily described than cases previously treated in childhood that then present with residual problems as adults.

On the other hand, patients who have had mainstream treatment of idiopathic congential clubfoot in the United States present with a variegated pattern of problems, as well as variable severity of each problem. This is because of the variable nature of the original clubfoot deformity and the wide variety of treatments used over the many decades and locations. Some of the patients presenting the deformity in late adulthood were treated solely by casting, whereas those presenting in early adulthood and early middle age have been more predominantly treated with surgical releases. The trend now favors more limited surgical intervention once again.[9,10]

There has been work done specifically on the subject of residual deformity of treated clubfoot. A study by Wei and colleagues[11] examined the results of talonavicular arthrodesis in patients with residual deformity after congenital clubfoot. They demonstrated satisfactory improvement of symptoms and radiographic improvement after surgery. Ramseier and colleagues[12] studied the outcome of triple arthrodesis to treat residual deformity in 7 adult patients who had been treated in childhood by Achilles lengthenings, soft tissue releases, and castings. They noted satisfactory clinical results, and improvement of deformity, but most patients had progression of adjacent joint arthritis both in the ankle and the midfoot postsurgically.

DIAGNOSIS

Physical examination should include evaluation of foot and ankle position in standing and non–weight bearing conditions. Examination includes range of motion, taking care to hold the ankle in maximum dorsiflexion while checking hindfoot motion, to prevent rocking motion of the plantarflexed talus in the mortise from simulating inversion and eversion.

Most relevant is the assessment of position and deformity of the ankle, the hindfoot, the transverse tarsal joints, and the forefoot.[13] The position of the heel in varus and valgus is the key. Assessment of equinus should separate its components occurring at the tibiotalar joint and at the talonavicular joint. The Coleman block test is the best known but not the only method to distinguish between the contribution to the cavus deformity of hindfoot varus and that to the plantarflexion of the first ray. Some patients have too much stiffness or equinus for the Coleman block test to be applied. The general principles of examination of the cavovarus foot apply in any case of this deformity. With the patient seated, it is possible to evaluate the flexibility of the hindfoot varus. With the ankle locked in dorsiflexion, if the heel can be passively corrected past neutral to a valgus position, then the subtalar joint and heel are not held in fixed varus. In that case, the primary component of the cavus deformity is located in the fixed plantarflexion of the first ray and the varus of the hindfoot is secondary and compensatory. However, in most cases of adult residual hindfoot varus, or cavovarus, the hindfoot is rigid and not flexible.

This is important in the determination of the appropriate surgical solution. If the first ray is rigidly plantarflexed, then the surgical correction must include dorsiflexion osteotomy of the first metatarsal. If the subtalar joint is even mildly or moderately flexible, then it is usually preferable to do an osteotomy of the calcaneus to improve the varus of the heel. If the subtalar joint is stiff, then subtalar arthrodesis, or triple arthrodesis, is not only more appropriate but also produces greater correction of the deformity.

Once the decision for surgical correction has been made, the choice between subtalar and triple arthrodeses depends on the deformity and stiffness at the transverse tarsal joints. This is determined according to not only the abduction and adduction at the talonavicular and calcaneocuboid joints but also the dorsiflexion of the talonavicular joint.

Radiographic examination must be composed of standing radiographs of the foot and the ankle. This may aid in the assessment of hindfoot varus. Radiographic representation of equinus is much less sensitive and accurate, and unless careful attention is paid to tibial position on the standing lateral view, it tends to underestimate the degree of clinical equinus.

CLINICAL PRESENTATION

It is certainly well known that incomplete correction and overcorrection can be hallmarks of congenital clubfoot and that the problems arising from this can present in childhood, as well as in adulthood. On the other hand, many surgeons have recognized the surprising ability of adolescents with congenital talipes equinovarus to participate, and excel, in a wide range of sporting activities through the middle school and high school years despite smaller foot and calf size and the profound weakness of the lower leg and ankle, which are hallmarks of clubfoot.

Than taking an approach that begins with specific treatments, we should examine the major problems with which these patients present. These problems include: overcorrection or valgus deformities, undercorrection or varus deformities, ankle and foot arthritis, and degenerative conditions of the ankle and hindfoot. The last category represents problems of the foot and ankle that are commensurate to the patient's age and may be exacerbated by, but not necessarily caused by, the underlying congenital deformity or its treatment.

These patients present with persistent new or recurrent pain. They are not necessarily recognizable as cases of failed surgical correction, neither over- nor undercorrection. Rather, many, if not most, patients have been considered treatment successes in childhood and adolescence. As is well recognized in the literature, the successful treatment of idiopathic congenital clubfoot does not result in a normal foot. Rather, it is to produce a foot that is reasonably plantigrade. Many of these patients present the deformity in adulthood because they experience a gradually diminishing tolerance of the residual deformity of the foot, or have increasing symptoms because of progressive arthritic change associated with the residual deformities of the ankle and hindfoot or both. Lastly, some present instead, or in addition, common degenerative conditions of the ankle and foot, which may be heightened by the underlying deformities. Examples include posterior tibial tendon dysfunction, subluxation and tears of the peroneal tendons, tendinosis of the Achilles tendon, and so forth.

Overcorrection

Overcorrection presents as the patient with a foot with hindfoot valgus, with or without pes planus (**Fig. 1**). Associated with this are symptoms of calcaneofibular impingement and radiographic findings of flattening of the dome of the talus. These patients are less likely to require surgical reconstruction and less likely to benefit from adult reconstruction than patients with undercorrection. Associated with the valgus deformity may be problems with the peroneal tendons that develop symptomatic tears as a result of calcaneofibular impingement. This is less likely and less common than peroneal pathology associated with varus deformity (**Fig. 2**).

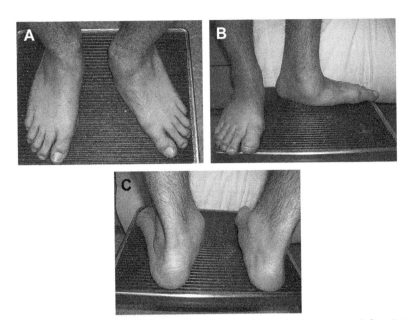

Fig. 1. (*A*) Previously treated clubfoot with overcorrection and severe valgus deformity seen from dorsally. (*B*) Valgus deformity from overcorrection of clubfoot with rocker deformity at the midfoot. (*C*) Same valgus deformity seen from posterior view.

The deformed talus, specifically the deformity of the talar dome, is particularly challenging because arthritic symptoms related to deformities of the talus both in cases of undercorrection and overcorrection may worsen with time, despite appropriate surgical intervention. The term "flat-top talus" frequently underdescribes the complex nature of the deformity of the talus, which not only has a flattened superior articular surface but also is abnormal in its overall morphology. These talar deformities may be nearly universal in these cases, although of varying degrees of severity. In common is the tendency to affect ankle and subtalar joints. This combined effect, usually expressed as symptoms of arthritis and deformity, complicates the treatment choices in advanced cases because arthrodesis at both levels is successful at eliminating pain

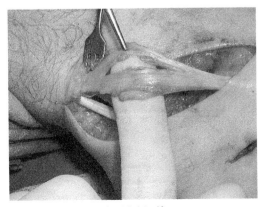

Fig. 2. Peroneal tendon tears associated with hindfoot varus.

and correcting deformity but at the cost of the already diminished residual range of motion, especially of the ankle.

Undercorrection

Undercorrection is more common in presentation of the adult sequelae of congenital clubfoot than overcorrection. It is unclear whether this is a reflection of an actual greater incidence of undercorrection than overcorrection or simply that varus deformities (undercorrection) are more likely to be symptomatic than valgus ones (overcorrection).

These patients have residual hindfoot varus, with or without residual equinus at the ankle. Each may exist to differing degrees (**Fig. 3**). In addition, there may be equinus and varus at the talonavicular joint as well. The challenge is to analyze each component of the deformity and to evaluate them separately to formulate a plan to address them.

Unlike children with recurrent deformity who can be treated with repeat soft tissue releases,[9,14] adults with symptomatic residual deformity require predominantly bony procedures with or without adjunct soft tissue balancing, of which the soft tissue procedures are secondary and the bony procedures are primary. The most common adjunct soft tissue procedures are Achilles lengthening, gastrocnemius recession, and plantar fascia release, followed by tendon procedures associated with correction of hammertoe and claw toe deformities.

ARTHRITIS

Arthritis of the ankle, subtalar, and talonavicular joints is common among these patients. One challenge is to distinguish arthritis as the cause of pain, separate from the issue of the deformity itself. The symptoms that can most clearly be attributed to varus deformities, apart from arthritic changes that may also be associated, are those that are the direct results of pressure caused by the deformity. Thus, pain over the lateral border of the foot, at the base of the fifth metatarsal would be caused

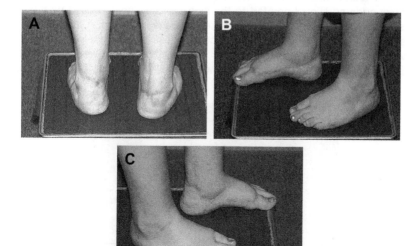

Fig. 3. (A) Bilateral hindfoot varus seen from posterior view. Note scars from posteromedial release done in infancy. (B & C) Medial and lateral views of both feet showing residual adduction of the forefoot, mild elevation of the first rays and fixed forefoot supination.

by the varus deformity. Pain under the head of the fifth metatarsal would also be caused by varus and exacerbated by equinus (**Fig. 4**).

Although most adult patients discussed here have radiographic evidence of arthritic changes of the ankle and/or hindfoot, the symptoms do not necessarily correspond to those radiographic findings. Usually, the symptoms are less severe than the radiographic changes, but the opposite can be true. Even more common is the lack of correlation between stiffness of the hindfoot and radiographic evidence of arthritis. Many, if not most, of these patients have loss of motion of the subtalar, talonavicular, and calcaneocuboid joints, which is not necessarily proportional to joint space narrowing or to the level of pain.

CONCURRENT DEGENERATIVE CONDITIONS

A challenge in hindfoot deformities is to identify whether pain localized to the lateral hindfoot is attributable to the subtalar joint, or to the peroneal tendons, or both. Hindfoot varus deformity predisposes to the development of peroneal tendon tears, especially of the peroneus brevis. The chronic subluxation of the peroneal tendons, which is induced by hindfoot varus, also mechanically leads to compression of the peroneus brevis against the distal fibula by the peroneus longus.

Tendinosis of the Achilles tendon, which is also a degenerative condition, is complicated by the scarring of Achilles tendon resulting from tendon lengthening at the time of the original surgical treatment.

Treatment

Treatment is initially conservative. The first level of treatment is use of a nonrigid, custom-molded, accommodative insole. This would typically be made of at least 2 different types of foams, of which 1 would be heat moldable. The mechanical properties and advantages of such insoles have been delineated in prior investigations.[15,16] Lateral wedges can be built into the insoles to counter the varus position of the hindfoot. An elevated lateral border of the insole that wraps around the base of the fifth metatarsal adds additional comfort to the high-pressure area caused by the varus. Insoles with rigid components are more likely to cause discomfort than to relieve it; the insoles should be shock absorbing because these feet themselves are rigid. The disadvantage of treatment with insoles is the limitation of footwear into which an adequate insole will fit. These footwears will be walking shoes, informal shoes, or

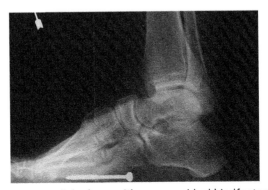

Fig. 4. Status post posteromedial release with severe residual hindfoot varus. Note the first ray plantar flexion. The severe hindfoot varus produced mechanical overload of the lateral border of the foot resulting in previously treated fifth metatarsal fracture.

athletic shoes. The recent advent in the popularity of shoes with curved soles has been an enormous boon to the treatment of numerous conditions of the foot and ankle. These are essentially popular and widely accepted versions of rocker-bottom shoes, without the unattractive moniker. The rocker-bottom effect of these shoes can be enhanced by the addition of a stiffening device made of carbon fiber or spring steel under the insole.

The second level of conservative treatment is the use of ankle-foot orthosis (AFO). The disadvantage of AFO is the reduced cosmesis, the bulk, and the limitation of foot-wear that will hold the AFO. However, this is outweighed by the advantages in mechanical control and pain relief both for the ankle and for the hindfoot.

The AFO can be either with a solid ankle or with an ankle hinge (short-articulated ankle-foot orthosis). The latter can have either an anterior or a posterior shell above the ankle. The solid AFO has the advantages of a slimmer profile, less bulk, and control of the tibiotalar joint. Both are best made and most comfortable when lined with plastazote foam. Modifications can be made to the AFO, which can compensate for equinus and varus (**Fig. 5D**). The use of the AFO is particularly effective for the pain of ankle and hindfoot arthritis in patients who elect nonsurgical treatment.

Surgical Reconstruction

One of the challenges of undercorrection is to recognize and separate the components of deformity occurring at the tibiotalar joint versus those occurring in the hind-foot, midfoot, and forefoot. The hindfoot deformities are somewhat easier to address through osteotomy or hindfoot arthrodesis, whereas the tibiotalar deformities are more difficult to address because they frequently represent a residual abnormality

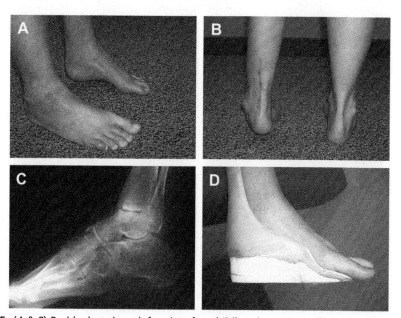

Fig. 5. (*A & B*) Residual equinus deformity after childhood posteromedial release as well as hindfoot varus. The heel does not touch the ground. (*C*) Lateral radiograph demonstrates the varus of the hindfoot, arthritic change in the tibiotalar joint and the mechanical block at the ankle preventing correction of the equinus. (*D*) Custom polypropylene AFO to control varus and with compensatory heel elevation to accommodate equinus.

in the morphology of the talus itself. If the pain at the level of the tibiotalar joint is severe, then arthrodesis is the preferred surgical intervention because it has a reliable result, is a durable construct, and can correct deformity as well as resolve pain.

Most of the patients with residual cavovarus or undercorrection have a component of equinus. This may be the result, in part, of a tight tendo Achilles tendon. However, these patients get only partial correction of the equinus deformity after a repeat tendo-Achilles lengthening because the talar dome deformity produces a mechanical block to dorsiflexion (see **Fig. 5**A–C). This mechanical block is a more important cause of equinus at the level of the ankle than recurrent soft tissue contracture in adults. Weakness of the triceps surae resulting from overlengthening the Achilles in childhood is associated with worse clinical results.[2] Also worth noting is the component of equinus at the talonavicular joint.

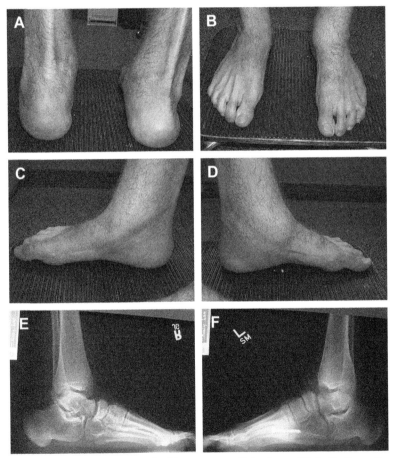

Fig. 6. (A) Bilateral clubfoot treated with posteromedial release. Clinically the patient has varus on the left and valgus on the right, as seen from posterior. (B) Antero posterior view the same. (C & D) Medial views of right and left feet, respectively. (E & F) Lateral radiographs of each foot. Note the residual abnormalities on both; the greater valgus on the right and the morphologic and arthritic changes on both feet. There is both change in the shape of the talus, abnormality in the talar dome, and deformity at the talar head at the interface with the navicular. Note the changes in shape of the navicular, cuboid, talus and calcaneus as well.

Cases of overcorrection less frequently require surgical correction in adults; the corollary is that there are fewer options for reconstruction. One is reconstruction of peroneal tendon tear that have occurred as a result of calcaneofibular impingement and the other is hindfoot arthrodesis if there is painful arthritis.

As noted earlier, the degree of arthritis radiographically does not necessarily correlate with the level of symptoms. Decisions for surgery should be made based primarily on the clinical symptoms. As illustrated in the case photos, the same patient who underwent bilateral soft tissue releases as an infant for clubfoot can present with 1 foot in varus and 1 in valgus (**Fig. 6**).

Attention must be paid to the deformity of the forefoot, and this is separately addressed in the course of surgical reconstruction. Forefoot deformity can be composed of different extremes, ranging from fixed forefoot supination (ie, elevation of the first ray [**Fig. 7**]) to fixed forefoot pronation (ie, rigid plantarflexion of the first ray [see **Fig. 6**D and **Fig. 4**]). Correction is addressed either through osteotomy of the first ray or through tarsometatarsal arthrodesis. The deformity of the first metatarsophalangeal (MTP) joint needs to be addressed at the same time. In the case of fixed elevation of the first ray, there is reciprocal plantarflexion of the first MTP joint and in fixed plantarflexion of the first ray, the opposite. Decisions for surgical reconstruction must be individualized according to the combination of specific deformities.

SUMMARY

One of the principles of treatment of these patients includes recognition that no one description of deformities applies to all cases of painful deformity in adults after

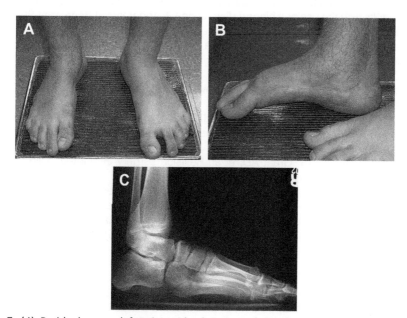

Fig. 7. (A) Residual varus deformity with elevation of the first ray seen from dorsally. (B) Medial view showing the first ray elevation and compensatory plantar flexion of the hallux. (C) Lateral radiograph demonstrating hindfoot varus, talar dome flattening, deformities of subtalar, talonavicular and calcaneo-cuboid joints; marked supination of the forefoot with severe first ray elevation.

childhood treatment of congenital clubfoot. There is a spectrum of the types of deformity and a range of severity among these that must be taken into account in the decision making regarding treatment.

Because so many of these patients have joint stiffness and because there is underlying bony deformity, it would be anticipated that these patients will develop progressive arthritis in the later decades of adult life. All of these are factors in the emphasis on arthrodesis as a surgical solution in the patients with advanced pain. Although the level of symptoms is very variable and ankle and hindfoot arthrodeses have the disadvantage of increasing mechanical stress and subsequent arthritis in the midfoot, arthrodesis and, to a lesser degree, osteotomy remain the mainstays of surgical reconstruction in the adult with painful deformity after treatment of congenital talipes equinovarus.

REFERENCES

1. Laaveg SJ, Ponseti IV. Long-term results of treatment of congenital club foot. J Bone Joint Surg Am 1980;62:23–31.
2. Cooper DM, Dietz FR. Treatment of idiopathic clubfoot a thirty-year follow-up note. J Bone Joint Surg Am 1995;77:1477–89.
3. Weinstein SL. Long-term follow-up of pediatric orthopaedic conditions. Natural history and outcomes of treatment. J Bone Joint Surg Am 2000;82(7):980–90.
4. Hutchins PM, Foster BK, Paterson DC, et al. Longterm results of early surgical release in clubfeet. J Bone Joint Surg Br 1985;67:791–9.
5. de la Huerta F. Correction of the neglected clubfoot by the Ilizarov method. Clin Orthop Relat Res 1994;301:89–93.
6. Oganesyan OV, Istomina IS, Kuzmin VI. Treatment of equinocavovarus deformity in adults with the use of a hinged distraction++ apparatus. J Bone Joint Surg Am 1996;78(4):546–56.
7. Salinas G, Chotigavanichaya C, Otsuka NY. A 30 year functional follow-up of a neglected congenital clubfoot in an adult: a case report. Foot Ankle Int 2000;21(12):1037–9.
8. Younger AS, Hansen ST Jr. Adult cavovarus foot. J Am Acad Orthop Surg 2005;13(5):302–15.
9. Morcuende JA, Dolan IA, Dietz FR, et al. Radical reduction in the rate of extensive corrective surgery for clubfoot using the Ponseti method. Pediatrics 2004;113(2):376–80.
10. Atar D, Lehman WB, Grant AD, et al. Revision surgery in clubfeet. Clin Orthop 1992;283:223–30.
11. Wei SY, Sullivan RJ, Davidson RS. Talo-navicular arthrodesis for residual midfoot deformities of a previously corrected clubfoot. Foot Ankle Int 2000;21(6):482–5.
12. Ramseier LE, Schoeniger R, Vienne P, et al. Treatment of late recurring idiopathic clubfoot deformity in adults. Acta Orthop Belg 2007;73(5):641–7.
13. Walling AK. The adult clubfoot (congenital pes cavus). Foot Ankle Clin 2008;13(2):307–14, vii.
14. Tarraf YN, Carroll NC. Analysis of the components of residual deformity in clubfeet presenting for reoperation. J Pediatr Orthop 1992;12:207–16.
15. Brodsky JW, Kourosh S, Stills M, et al. Objective evaluation of insert material for diabetic and athletic footwear. Foot Ankle 1988;9(3):111–6.
16. Brodsky JW, Pollo FE, Cheleuitte D, et al. Physical properties, durability, and energy- dissipation function of dual-density orthotic materials in insoles for diabetic patients. Foot Ankle Int 2007;28(8):880–9.

Idiopathic Toe Walking and Contractures of the Triceps Surae

Matthew C. Solan, FRCS (Tr&Orth)[a],*,
Julie Kohls-Gatzoulis, FRCS (Tr&Orth)[a],
Michael M. Stephens, MSc (Bioeng), FRCSI[b]

KEYWORDS

• Idiopathic toe walking • Achilles tendon • Gastrocnemius

This article examines the evidence for the management of children who have idiopathic toe walking and reviews the literature on surgery for the lengthening of a calf contracture.

IDIOPATHIC TOE WALKING
Presentation

Toe walking is a common feature in immature gait and is considered normal up to 3 years of age. As walking ability improves, initial contact is made with the heel. Toe-walker will stand out as different once heel-strike is achieved by most of their peers. This difference gives rise to parental concern. Therefore, toe-walkers are often referred at the 3 years of age.

For children who persistently walk on their toes present, orthopedic surgeons must consider whether there is an underlying cause for the observed gait (ie, an abnormality of the musculoskeletal or neurologic system) or the toe walking is idiopathic.

The second issue relates to management of the child and their parents. Because idiopathic means that no cause is identifiable, the gait may improve spontaneously. Surgeons therefore must consider whether long-term problems are likely, should any treatment be recommended, and, if so, whether surgery plays a role.

Differential Diagnosis and Pathophysiology

Idiopathic toe walking is a diagnosis that can only be reached once other causes for a similar pattern of gait have been excluded. Duchenne muscular dystrophy and

[a] Department of Trauma and Orthopaedic Surgery, Royal Surrey County Hospital, Egerton Road, Guildford, Surrey GU2 5XX,UK
[b] Department of Orthopaedic Surgery, Children's University Hospital, Temple Street, Dublin 1, Ireland
* Corresponding author.
E-mail address: matthewsolan1@aol.com

Foot Ankle Clin N Am 15 (2010) 297–307
doi:10.1016/j.fcl.2010.01.002
1083-7515/10/$ – see front matter © 2010 Elsevier Inc. All rights reserved.

foot.theclinics.com

abnormal psychological profiles must be considered.[1,2] In practice, however, the most difficult distinction is between mild cerebral palsy with diplegia (CP) and idiopathic toe walking (ITW). On clinical examination, these can be differentiated by the normal resting muscle tone in patients who have ITW. In general, children who have CP have tight hamstrings and normal calf muscle tone. Children who have ITW who present young and have no calf contracture are best considered as having overactive triceps surae. Whether persistent toe walking results in true shortening of the calf over time is uncertain.

Children who have ITW have normal hamstring length, and this is often used to distinguish these groups clinically. However, it is not reliable, and therefore gait analysis has been used to define the differences.[1–3]

In the CP group, Hicks and colleagues[2] showed that any abnormality observed at the ankle is not the primary deformity. Instead, the equinus is secondary to knee posture consequent on contracture of the hamstrings. A group of normal children, when asked to walk on their toes, showed kinematics identical to the ITW subjects.[3]

When muscular dystrophy is suspected, the history may show a period of normal gait before the onset of toe walking. The diagnosis is confirmed through muscle biopsy. In one study, investigators performed a muscle biopsy on 25 patients undergoing treatment for ITW (calf release or application of cast under general anesthesia), with results showing mild abnormalities and an increase in the proportion of type 1 muscle fibers. The investigators postulated that this was caused by a subtle neuropathy and drew parallels with the findings in patients who have talipes.[4]

Management of Idiopathic Toe Walking

Management of children who have idiopathic toe walking is controversial. If the natural history were fully understood, then clinical decision making would be easier. Predicting whether an individual's gait will spontaneously improve to allow heel strike at initial contact is not possible currently.

Based on the assumption that ITW often improves without intervention, reassurance alone is one treatment option commonly used. Parents should understand that Foot and Ankle Surgeons caring for adult patients are not often faced with symptoms directly related to a persistence of childhood toe walking. Furthermore, these symptoms can be managed on their own merits, when necessary, in adulthood.

However, recognition is increasing that a wide variety of pathologies are associated with longstanding calf contracture.[5] Gastrocnemius tightness has been implicated in many foot and ankle disorders in the adult population, including plantar fasciitis, Achilles tendinopathy, painful pes planus, tibialis posterior dysfunction, forefoot overload, and diabetic pressure ulcers.[5–10]

Published Literature on the Management of Idiopathic Toe Walking

The literature includes many reviews of small groups of children. Some have long-term follow-up, but the studies are varied making interpretation difficult. Only one series remains that has a long follow-up and large patient number.[1]

Some studies include patients both with and without loss of ankle dorsiflexion on physical examination. One series included only patients who had mild deformity (all managed nonoperatively).[11] When examined, all children in this cohort could achieve a plantigrade ankle. Other authors treated children differently according to whether the contracture was confined to the gastrocnemius or present when the knee was extended and flexed.[12]

Treatment without surgery

Hirsch and Wagner[11] reported on the outcome of long-term follow-up in 14 children, all managed nonoperatively. Although 16 patients were identified as having ITW, 2 were excluded from the study because they underwent surgery at another institution. The age at presentation ranged from 3 to 9 years, and length of follow-up ranged from 7 to 21 years. Of the 14 children, 8 had a positive family history. All 14 were managed with a passive stretching regimen, and 5 underwent a period of casting (<4 weeks) and then physiotherapy with or without night splints. None of the children had a fixed contracture of the calf either at presentation or at long-term follow-up, and 11 no longer exhibited toe walking. Of the 3 that still did, 2 had mild persistent symptoms that could be attributed to the persistence of abnormal gait. The authors concluded that ITW is a condition that usually corrects spontaneously and that any surgical treatment should be reserved for cases showing calf contracture.

Patients treated with casting, followed by surgery in recalcitrant cases

Stott and colleagues[13] reviewed another small cohort of patients at 5 to 15 years follow-up. This study involved 13 patients, all managed initially with stretches and casting. Of these patients, 7 still exhibited toe walking and were treated surgically. Unlike the patients reviewed by Hirsch and Wagner,[11] this group had all reached skeletal maturity at time of review. Clinical assessment, gait analysis, and calf strength were all reported. None of the subjects expressed dissatisfaction with the treatment they had received, although two patients reported a tendency to still walk on their toes. Passive ankle dorsiflexion was reduced in relation to population norms. All patients except one showed reduced measurements for peak ankle dorsiflexion during gait analysis. Preoperative gait analysis was not available. Only one patient showed ankle plantarflexion at initial contact. Calf strength was not significantly different between operatively and nonoperatively managed groups.

Hemo and colleagues[14] reviewed 15 children treated with Achilles tendon lengthening at a mean of 1 year postoperatively. They found that nonoperative measures failed to correct the problem in 12 patients. and the other 3 had pronounced equinus deformity at presentation and were considered to have a very poor chance of improving with nonoperative treatment. Gait analysis was conducted before and after surgical treatment.

Surgery to lengthen the Achilles tendon was performed percutaneously in 3 patients and as an open procedure in the other 12. The average age at surgery was 9 years (range, 4–13 years). Mean follow-up was 2.9 years. Mean ankle dorsiflexion with the knee extended improved from –7.5° preoperatively to 11.6° postoperatively. Improvement in dorsiflexion was seen when the knee was bent from a mean of –0.3° to 15°.

Plantarflexion strength (measured according to ability to perform 10 toe raises) was normal before and after surgery. Sagittal plane kinematics showed that dorsiflexion improved and overlengthening did not occur. In fact, calculation of power at push-off showed a postoperative increase, although this did not reach statistical significance and did not reach normal levels. Preoperatively, seven patients showed knee recurvatum during stance phase, and six of these improved postoperatively.

The authors concluded that careful Achilles lengthening is successful in idiopathic toe walkers when nonoperative management failed. They caution against surgery in patients who have no fixed ankle equinus deformity.

McMulkin and colleagues[12] reviewed the results of 14 patients who had pre- and postoperative gait analysis whose treatment involved gastrocnemius release (Vulpius) or Achilles tendon lengthening (6 percutaneous and 1 open). The Silfverskiold test was the basis for the decision to lengthen just the gastrocnemius or the Achilles tendon.

Surgery improved ankle dorsiflexion in stance and swing phase, and reduced the abnormal pelvic tilt that was seen particularly in the group that required Achilles lengthening (as opposed to the less-severely equinus group treated with a gastrocnemius release). External rotation of the hip and the foot-progression angle was noted preoperatively and did not alter after surgery.

Treatment with surgery, casting, or reassurance

Eastwood and colleagues[1] reviewed 136 patients from a cohort of 185 cases referred over a 22-year period. Follow-up ranged from 2 to 22 years. The review included three treatment groups, although like other series, the indications for different management strategies are not well defined. Patients were managed with reassurance and no further treatment advised; serial below-knee walking casts for 6 weeks; or surgical lengthening.

Results show no difference in outcome between the group treated with casting and the group offered no treatment. The authors conclude that casting does not improve the natural history of the condition. A normal gait was seen in 12% of patients who underwent casting and 22% of those in the observation group. In both groups, 49% of patients reported no improvement in gait.

The surgical group were a mean of 2 years older than the children in the other two groups. Outcome was better with a more normal gait, both subjectively (72%) and objectively (37%). Statistical comparison with the other two groups was not made because the age difference was considered to be a potentially important confounding variable. Nevertheless, the authors conclude that "it is likely that the outcome after surgical intervention is an improvement on the natural history."[1]

SUMMARY OF LITERATURE REVIEW

Review of the literature leaves surgeons with many unanswered questions:

Does idiopathic toe walking matter when the number of patients presenting as adults with problems directly attributed to ITW is very small? If ITW is untreated does a contracture develop over time? Does the natural history vary according to the presence of a contracture? If so, should there be a distinction between idiopathic toe-walkers (who have an unexplained contracture) and habitual toe-walkers (who have sufficient dorsiflexion of the ankle to achieve a plantigrade stance)? When evidence of a contracture is present, does it matter whether it is occurs in the whole triceps surae or is confined to the gastrocnemius? Is the surgical outcome after gastrocnemius lengthening better than after (open or percutaneous) Achilles tendon lengthening?

Based on the best evidence from the published literature, limited conclusions can be drawn:

The natural history of ITW suggests spontaneous improvement but not that the gait to become completely normal.
The condition usually persists despite nonoperative treatments, including casting.
Non-operative treatments offer no improvement in outcome over observation alone.
Surgery has a low complication rate but only produces an improved, rather than normal, gait. Surgery may be best reserved for cases with a demonstrable contracture. Where surgery is chosen, a gastrocnemius release may be preferable to Achilles lengthening.

CALF CONTRACTURE
Pathomechanics and Surgery

The exact amount of ankle dorsiflexion required for normal gait is controversial, but it is generally accepted that ankle dorsiflexion past neutral (<10°) is required. During terminal stance phase, maximal ankle dorsiflexion occurs just before the heel lifts from the ground. At this moment of maximal ankle dorsiflexion, the knee is extended (stretching the gastrocnemius) and the foot supinates to create a rigid structure for leverage.

In individuals who have a tight calf, several compensatory mechanisms can be observed:

Early heel off, causing increased pressure under the forefoot. The resultant forefoot overload is implicated in many different problems that affect the adult foot.

Shifting the center of mass forward relative to the foot, which can be accomplished by increasing lumbar lordosis, hip flexion, or knee recurvatum (**Fig 1**).

Subtalar joint pronation (**Fig 2**). With the transverse tarsal joint unlocked, dorsiflexion occurs through the talonavicular and calcaneocuboid joints. This mechanism increases strain in the tibialis posterior tendon and spring ligament. Gastrocnemius contracture has been implicated in tibialis posterior dysfunction.[15]

External rotation of the leg to shorten the lever arm of the foot.

A static cadaver model showed that isolated gastrocnemius tightness can increase mid- and forefoot pressure at the end of stance phase. Isolated gastrocnemius tightness produces the same changes as combined gastrocnemius–soleus tightness.[15] If the contracture is isolated to the gastrocnemius, then surgical lengthening is only required for this portion of the calf musculature.

The Silfverskiold test is used to distinguish between contractures that are predominantly in the gastrocnemius and those that affect both the gastrocnemius and soleus. The proximal attachment of the gastrocnemius to the posterior surface of the femoral condyles causes this muscle to be tight when the knee is extended. When the knee is flexed, the gastrocnemius relaxes. Therefore, a loss of ankle dorsiflexion that is evident when the knee is flexed must affect the soleus and gastrocnemius. If the

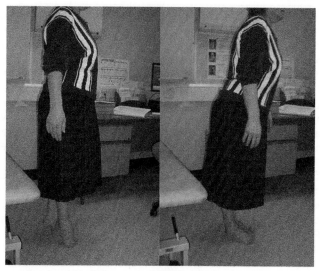

Fig. 1. Compensating for calf contracture – coronal plane.

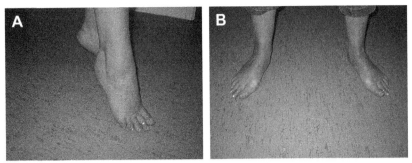

Fig. 2. (A) Compensating for calf contracture, preferred posture. (B) Heel–ground contact only possible with pronation and wide stance.

contracture is present with the knee fully extended but improves with knee flexion, then the soleus is not contributing to the contracture, and the calf contracture is limited to the gastrocnemius (**Fig 3**).

Nonoperative Treatment

The role of physiotherapy and serial casting in the treatment of ITW is discussed earlier. Eastwood and colleagues,[1] who published the largest review, found no difference between patients managed with serial casts for 6 weeks and those offered no treatment.

In contrast, for adult patients whose plantar fasciitis and Achilles tendinopathy are managed with gastrocnemius stretches, the results are impressive[6,16] in terms of improving gastrocnemius tightness and heel pain. Experiments have also shown that increased tension in the tendoachilles leads to increased plantar fascia tension and strain,[17,18] offering an explanation for why stretching the gastrocnemius improves heel pain. No published literature support the anecdotal evidence that casting produces lasting improvement of calf contracture in adults.

Operative Treatment

When surgery is considered for treating calf contracture, the technique must be appropriate for the type of contracture. The Silfverskiold test[19] allows surgeons to determine whether the contracture is in the gastrocnemius and soleus or confined to the gastrocnemius portion of the triceps surae.

Cadaver studies have shown that the degree to which forefoot pressures increase is similar when force is increased through either the whole triceps or just the gastrocnemius.[15] Surgical release of the Achilles tendon is associated with a risk for weakness from overlengthening. A lengthy rehabilitation period is also associated with casting. For these reasons, when the Silfverskiold test confirms that the contracture is confined to the gastrocnemius, release of just this portion of the calf should be preferred.[15]

Surgical Release

Vulpius and Stoffel,[20] Silfverskiöld,[19] and Strayer[21] published the pioneering work on gastrocnemius release. Many different releases have now been described. Classifying the anatomic level of the gastrocnemius–soleus complex is useful when the release is performed (**Fig 4**).[22]

Silfverskiöld[19] described an operation that releases the heads of the gastrocnemius from their origin on the femur (level five), but reported problems with postoperative knee swelling.

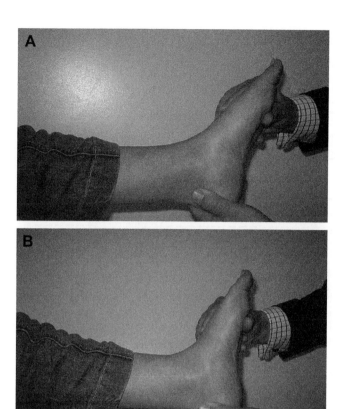

Fig. 3. The Silfverskiold test, (A) knee extended and (B) knee flexed.

The Bauman procedure divides the aponeurosis covering the deep (anterior) surface of the gastrocnemius (level four).[22] The procedure is performed through a medial incision and places the saphenous nerve and greater saphenous vein at risk. The surgical dissection is deep, necessitating general anesthesia. An assistant is needed for retraction so the undersurface of the gastrocnemius muscle can be reached.

Strayer[21] described an open release at the gastrocnemius insertion onto the tendoachilles (level three). Strayer allowed the gastrocnemius to retract and then he reattached the muscle more proximally. The course and formation of the sural nerve have five common variations,[23] and operations at this level place it at risk. In addition, the sural nerve can be superficial, deep, or closely applied to the fascia at this level.[24] After a Strayer release, the patient is immobilized for at least 2 weeks.[25,26] This is another disadvantage of a surgical release at this level. Poor wound cosmesis has also been reported.[24,26] The Strayer release has been associated with a 6% overall rate of complication. Furthermore, 5% of patients complained of poor wound cosmesis and 3% had nerve damage. The nerve damage to the sural or saphenous nerve was transient in most patients, but transection of the nerve leading to complex regional pain syndrome was reported.

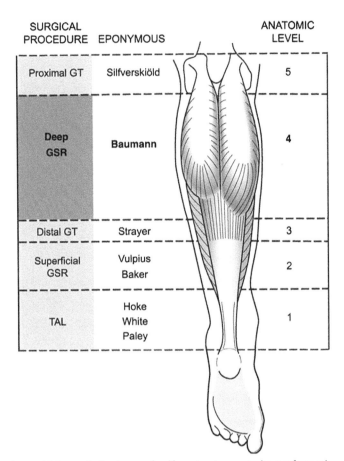

SURGICAL PROCEDURE	EPONYMOUS	ANATOMIC LEVEL
Proximal GT	Silfverskiöld	5
Deep GSR	Baumann	4
Distal GT	Strayer	3
Superficial GSR	Vulpius Baker	2
TAL	Hoke White Paley	1

Fig. 4. Levels at which surgical release of calf contracture may be performed.

Endoscopic Strayer release was recently described.[27–30] The sural nerve is at risk, with neuropraxia reported in 3 of 18 patients in one series.[29] The aponeurosis at this level is a thick structure, and difficulties using the shaver to release it completely have been reported. In one cadaver study, only half of the specimens examined after completion of the procedure had been fully released.[30]

The Vulpius procedure (level two) is often used for children who have spastic diplegia. In this procedure, the external aponeurosis of the gastrocnemius and the underlying superficial aponeurosis of soleus are sectioned transversely just distal to the gastrocnemius muscle belly.[20,31] The Vulpius procedure therefore must lengthen the gastrocnemius and soleus.

Although no nomenclature is applied, Sammarco and colleagues[32] describes the effects of a gastrocnemius lengthening at level two and found a 5% incidence of paraesthesia in the sural nerve distribution and 5% incidence of complaints related to the wound.

Level one is the Achilles tendon itself. Z-lengthening or triple-cut techniques may be performed either open or percutaneously. Cadaver work has shown that percutaneous techniques are unreliable[33] and risk damage to adjacent nerves.[34] Open surgery is recommended.[33] Wound healing and weakness are both potential complications with significant associated morbidity.[35]

Level four is the ideal level to perform an isolated release of the gastrocnemius when the contracture is mild or moderate. The lengthening is restricted to the tight gastrocnemius aponeurosis; no damage occurs to either the insertion or the origin of the muscle, and the risk for neurologic complication is extremely low.

European authors[36,37] have reported a simple and safe gastrocnemius release in level four. When the contracture is pronounced, both heads can be released through a single popliteal crease incision under general anesthesia. Because the medial head has been noted to be the source of most of the gastrocnemius tightness, less severe cases can be treated with a proximal release of the aponeurosis of the medial head in isolation. This procedure is safe and can be performed under local anesthetic with sedation (in adults). Furthermore, patients mobilize immediately after surgery without the need for a protective plaster. The wound heals very well with none of the complications seen with the Strayer[37,38] procedure.

Results and Complications of Gastrocnemius Lengthening

Short-term reports show that ankle dorsiflexion with the knee extended improves to the same amount achieved with the knee flexed.[25] No studies confirm that this correction is maintained over time, and limited literature has examined whether a change in muscle strength occurs with the various lengthening operations described.

With the Strayer release, the possibility of weakness is a concern.[39] The benchmarks for Medical Research Council power grading for the gastrocnemius–soleus complex are as follows: 5/5 power permits 30 single heel rises; 4/5 power permits 5, and 3/5 power permits one single heel rise.[39,40] However, this is controversial because other work has shown that the maximal number of single heel rises individuals can perform depends on the their age and gender.[41]

Attempts to measure the ability to perform a single heel rise after Strayer release have been challenging, because many patients also underwent simultaneous surgery for other foot pathology (eg, midfoot arthrosis treated with fusion).[26] The same authors documented that all patients who had an isolated Strayer release were able to perform five single heel rises at 6 months postoperatively.[26] No prospective data compare strength before and after release. When comparing peak torque with the normal side after surgery, Sammarco and colleagues[32] found it to be on average 74% of the unaffected side, with a trend toward strength improvement 18 months after surgery as opposed to 18 months before surgery.

Research has been performed on the Vulpius lengthening and its affect on the medial head of the gastrocnemius in children who have CP.[31] Using ultrasound to assess the medial head of the gastrocnemius preoperatively, 7 weeks postoperative, and 1 year after surgery, muscle volume actually increased in most limbs at 1 year, but the difference was not statistically significant. After Vulpius lengthening, the medial gastrocnemius muscle length was reduced despite improvement in ankle dorsiflexion. The lengthening was therefore achieved through the external aponeurosis of the gastrocnemius, and the gastrocnemius belly itself actually shortened. Muscle power was not measured in this study.[42]

Summary of Surgery

There is increasing recognition that adult foot pathologies are associated with gastrocnemius shortening. The Silfverskiold test determines whether the equinus deformity is confined to the gastrocnemius. When a stretching program, supervised by a physiotherapist, fails to produce sufficient improvement, surgical release may be considered. Release of gastrocnemius alone is associated with less risk for complication and a shorter rehabilitation, and therefore should be preferred when the

Silfverskiold test confirms an isolated contracture of the gastrocnemius. These principles are applicable to adult and pediatric populations.

REFERENCES

1. Eastwood DM, Menelaus MB, Dickens DR, et al. Idiopathic toe-walking: does treatment alter the natural history? J Pediatr Orthop B 2000;9:47.
2. Hicks R, Durinick N, Gage JR. Differentiation of idiopathic toe-walking and cerebral palsy. J Pediatr Orthop 1988;8:160.
3. Kelly IP, Jenkinson A, Stephens M, et al. The kinematic patterns of toe-walkers. J Pediatr Orthop 1997;17:478.
4. Handelsman JE, Badalamente MA. Neuromuscular studies in clubfoot. J Pediatr Orthop 1981;1:23.
5. DiGiovanni CW, Kuo R, Tejwani N, et al. Isolated gastrocnemius tightness. J Bone Joint Surg Am 2002;84A:962.
6. Fahlstrom M, Jonsson P, Lorentzon R, et al. Chronic Achilles tendon pain treated with eccentric calf-muscle training. Knee Surg Sports Traumatol Arthrosc 2003; 11:327.
7. Ohberg L, Lorentzon R, Alfredson H. Eccentric training in patients with chronic Achilles tendinosis: normalised tendon structure and decreased thickness at follow up. Br J Sports Med 2004;38:8.
8. Reyolds NL, Worrell TW. Chronic Achilles peritendonitis: etiology, pathophysiology and treatment. J Orthop Sports Phys Ther 1991;13:171.
9. Riddle DL, Pulisic M, Pidcoe P, et al. Risk factors for Plantar fasciitis: a matched case-control study. J Bone Joint Surg Am 2003;85A:872.
10. Rompe JD, Furia J, Maffulli N. Eccentric loading compared with shock wave treatment for chronic insertional Achilles tendinopathy. A randomized, controlled trial. J Bone Joint Surg Am 2008;90:52.
11. Hirsch G, Wagner B. The natural history of idiopathic toe-walking: a long-term follow-up of fourteen conservatively treated children. Acta Paediatr 2004;93:196.
12. McMulkin ML, Baird GO, Caskey PM, et al. Comprehensive outcomes of surgically treated idiopathic toe walkers. J Pediatr Orthop 2006;26:606.
13. Stott NS, Walt SE, Lobb GA, et al. Treatment for idiopathic toe-walking: results at skeletal maturity. J Pediatr Orthop 2004;24:63.
14. Hemo Y, Macdessi SJ, Pierce RA, et al. Outcome of patients after Achilles tendon lengthening for treatment of idiopathic toe walking. J Pediatr Orthop 2006;26:336.
15. Aronow MS, Diaz-Doran V, Sullivan RJ, et al. The effect of triceps surae contracture force on plantar foot pressure distribution. Foot Ankle Int 2006;27:43.
16. Alfredson H, Lorentzon R. Chronic Achilles tendinosis: recommendations for treatment and prevention. Sports Med 2000;29:135.
17. Carlson RE, Fleming LL, Hutton WC. The biomechanical relationship between the tendoachilles, plantar fascia and metatarsophalangeal joint dorsiflexion angle. Foot Ankle Int 2000;21:18.
18. Erdemir A, Hamel AJ, Fauth AR, et al. Dynamic loading of the plantar aponeurosis in walking. J Bone Joint Surg Am 2004;86-A:546.
19. Silfverskiold N. Reduction of the uncrossed two-joint muscles of the leg to one joint muscles in spastic conditions. Acta Chir Scand 1924;56:315.
20. Vulpius O, Stoffel A. Orthopadishe Operationslehre. Stuttgart, Germany: Verlag von Ferdinand Enke; 1913 [in German].
21. Strayer LM Jr. Recession of the gastrocnemius; an operation to relieve spastic contracture of the calf muscles. J Bone Joint Surg Am 1950;32A:671.

22. Herzenberg JE, Lamm BM, Corwin C, et al. Isolated recession of the gastrocnemius muscle: the Baumann procedure. Foot Ankle Int 2007;28:1154.
23. Aktan Ikiz ZA, Ucerler H, Bilge O. The anatomic features of the sural nerve with an emphasis on its clinical importance. Foot Ankle Int 2005;26:560.
24. Pinney SJ, Sangeorzan BJ, Hansen ST Jr. Surgical anatomy of the gastrocnemius recession (Strayer procedure). Foot Ankle Int 2004;25:247.
25. Pinney SJ, Hansen ST Jr, Sangeorzan BJ. The effect on ankle dorsiflexion of gastrocnemius recession. Foot Ankle Int 2002;23:26.
26. Rush SM, Ford LA, Hamilton GA. Morbidity associated with high gastrocnemius recession: retrospective review of 126 cases. J Foot Ankle Surg 2006;45:156.
27. Barrett SL, Jarvis J. Equinus deformity as a factor in forefoot nerve entrapment: treatment with endoscopic gastrocnemius recession. J Am Podiatr Med Assoc 2005;95:464.
28. DiDomenico LA, Adams HB, Garchar D. Endoscopic gastrocnemius recession for the treatment of gastrocnemius equinus. J Am Podiatr Med Assoc 2005;95:410.
29. Saxena A, Widtfeldt A. Endoscopic gastrocnemius recession: preliminary report on 18 cases. J Foot Ankle Surg 2004;43:302.
30. Tashjian RZ, Appel AJ, Banerjee R, et al. Endoscopic gastrocnemius recession: evaluation in a cadaver model. Foot Ankle Int 2003;24:607.
31. Fry NR, Gough M, McNee AE, et al. Changes in the volume and length of the medial gastrocnemius after surgical recession in children with spastic diplegic cerebral palsy. J Pediatr Orthop 2007;27:769.
32. Sammarco GJ, Bagwe MR, Sammarco VJ, et al. The effects of unilateral gastrocsoleus recession. Foot Ankle Int 2006;27:508.
33. Hoefnagels EM, Waites MD, Belkoff SM, et al. Percutaneous Achilles tendon lengthening: a cadaver-based study of failure of the triple hemisection technique. Acta Orthop 2007;78:808.
34. Salamon ML, Pinney SJ, Van Bergeyk A, et al. Surgical anatomy and accuracy of percutaneous Achilles tendon lengthening. Foot Ankle Int 2006;27:411.
35. Delp SL, Statler K, Carroll NC. Preserving plantar flexion strength after surgical treatment for contracture of the triceps surae: a computer simulation study. J Orthop Res 1995;13:96.
36. Barouk LS, Barouk P, Toulec E. Resulltats de la liberation Proximale des Gastrocnemiens. Etude Prospective in Symposium Brieveté des Gastrocnemiens, Journées de Printemps SFMCP-AFCP. Toulouse, France: Med Chir Pied 2006;22:151 [in French].
37. Kohls-Gatzoulis JA, Solan M. Results of proximal medial gastrocnemius release. J Bone Joint Surg Br 2009;91B:361.
38. Barouk LS, Barouk P. Brièveté des gastrocnémiens. In: Compte rendu du symposium n°3, Journées de Printemps SFMCP-AFCP. Toulouse, France: 2006. p. 22 [in French].
39. Mann RA. RE: the effect on ankle dorsiflexion of gastrocsoleus recession, Pinney SJ, et al., Foot Ankle Int. 23(1):26–29, 2002. Foot Ankle Int 2003;24:726.
40. Perry J. Gait analysis—normal and pathological function. Thorofare (NJ): Stack; 1992.
41. Jan MH, Chai HM, Lin YF, et al. Effects of age and sex on the results of an ankle plantar-flexor manual muscle test. Phys Ther 2005;85:1078.
42. Baddar A, Granata K, Damiano DL, et al. Ankle and knee coupling in patients with spastic diplegia: effects of gastrocnemius-soleus lengthening. J Bone Joint Surg Am 2002;84A:736.

Management of the Flexible Flat Foot in the Child: A Focus on the Use of Osteotomies for Correction

John Y. Kwon, MD[a],*, Mark S. Myerson, MD[b]

KEYWORDS

• Pes planus • Flat foot deformity • Pediatric • Osteotomy

Pes planus, commonly referred as flat foot, is a combination of foot and ankle deformities. Along with the loss of the medial longitudinal arch, the heel is in various degrees of valgus alignment and the subtalar joint is generally incongruent. The midtarsal joints are abducted with supination of the forefoot. The talar head becomes prominent medially with plantar subluxation and as the navicular moves off the talar head, it becomes progressively uncovered. A valgus deformity of the tibiotalar joint can also be present, the result of chronic compression of the lateral epiphysis, adding to the valgus deformity of the hindfoot. There is no generic deformity, and marked variability not only in the location but also the severity is often present. Some patients may exhibit no abduction of the transverse tarsal joint at all, sometimes there is severe heel valgus, and at times there are combinations of these.

Often these children are asymptomatic, and the flat foot deformity is brought to the attention of a specialist due to the parent's concerns for underlying pathology and future impairment. It is critical that the treating surgeon understand normal variation from true pathology, as well as conditions that have a benign natural history versus those that may lead to significant disability if left untreated. A systematic method for evaluation is required, starting with determination of whether the foot is rigid or flexible. Many conditions that may cause rigid flat foot such as congenital vertical talus, tarsal coalitions, and accessory navicular often follow well-established guidelines for treatment, and are not discussed in this article. The treatment of the flexible flat

[a] Department of Orthopaedic Surgery, Harvard Medical School, Massachusetts General Hospital, Boston, MA 02114, USA
[b] Institute for Foot and Ankle Reconstruction at Mercy, Mercy Medical Center, 301 St Paul Place, Baltimore, MD 21201, USA
* Corresponding author.
E-mail address: johnkwonmd@gmail.com

Foot Ankle Clin N Am 15 (2010) 309–322
doi:10.1016/j.fcl.2010.02.001
1083-7515/10/$ – see front matter © 2010 Elsevier Inc. All rights reserved.

foot.theclinics.com

foot, whether painless or painful, requires considerable insight by the surgeon to avoid undue treatment of a benign process but also to avoid neglecting pathology with the potential for disability in adulthood. Is this art or science? Perhaps a bit of both, because there are few well-defined features of the flexible flat foot in the child that determine the need for surgical intervention. One must begin with the assumption that before initiating any treatment, the child should be symptomatic. There is no evidence whatsoever that the use of an orthotic support will change the structure of the arch of the growing foot; however, orthoses certainly should be used if the child is symptomatic, and with some expectation of success. When the child has persistent symptoms, the issue becomes more clouded, because activity will determine the need for subsequent treatment. However, what should one do with a child who has severe flat foot deformity but is entirely asymptomatic? Should one proceed with orthoses, or should one counsel the family on the potential benefits of surgery? There are certain children who are inevitably going to become more symptomatic as an adult, but it is understandably difficult to predict exactly who will be more symptomatic with increasing deformity and who will remain asymptomatic. Perhaps there is a "feel" to this, and one can anticipate that certain deformities will inevitably worsen and there-fore require surgery. Common sense clearly supports the indication for a simple procedure, such as an arthroereisis or an osteotomy, performed in the young child as opposed to an arthrodesis in older adolescence or adulthood as the foot becomes more rigid. This approach too is supported in the literature, and these and other issues are discussed in this article.

BACKGROUND

It is important to realize that we are all born with a flat foot. The normal infant foot is devoid of any recognizable arch and is instead filled with abundant fatty tissue. The full development of the normal arch typically occurs around age 5 years but can occur up to the first decade of life. Staheli and colleagues[1] demonstrated that flat foot is normal in infants and common in children. Similarly, Gould and colleagues[2] demon-strated that some level of pes planus was present in all of the toddlers in his study looking at arch development. However, the processes that result in development of the normal arch versus retention of a flat foot deformity into adulthood are not well understood and the natural history is not known.

Several researchers have demonstrated the increased prevalence of flat foot defor-mity in shod populations. Rao and Joseph[3] studied 2300 children, concluding that flat foot deformity was more often associated with closed toe shoes and less so with sandal/slipper wear and unshod feet. Sachithanandam and Joseph[4] studied 1846 adult persons in India and similarly found the incidence of flat foot to be significantly higher in those that wore shoes before the age of 6 years, suggesting a detrimental association between shoe wear and flat foot. Finally, Harris and Beath,[5] who studied 3600 Canadian recruits, determined that flat foot was not a cause of disability and foot pain in the adult, and suggested that flat foot deformity was normal along a spectrum of normal arch height.

HISTORY AND EXAMINATION

One needs adequate information from the child or parent to determine whether the flat foot deformity is painful or pain free. This population can range from toddlers who cannot reliably participate in history taking to adolescents who may downplay their symptomatology. Therefore, it is important to elicit additional history from the parents. The history should include pain location (if any), intensity, and alleviating/aggravating factors, a thorough documentation of any medical comorbidities (including other orthopedic conditions), birth history, age of walking, and attainment of developmental milestones. A history of trauma or recurrent ankle sprains should be specifically questioned. Particularly important in the overall decision making are the limitations during activities of daily living, recreational activities, and sports. The effect of shoe wear of various types should be determined.

Given the association of flat foot with other orthopedic conditions (including torsional abnormalities of the lower extremity), all pediatric patients should be examined with complete visualization of the unclothed lower extremities. Compliance with physical examination often depends on the age of the patient. For younger children, simple observation of the barefoot child in the examination room can elicit useful data. Similarly, the parents can be asked to participate in the physical examination for younger children who may be fearful of examination by the physician. For all patients the foot and ankle should be examined with the patient standing and sitting, as a flat foot deformity may not be apparent in the absence of weight bearing. Range of motion should be determined, with special attention paid to Achilles contractures. As the hindfoot deforms into a valgus position the Achilles complex is not only deviated laterally but shortened as well, leading to contracture.

Flexibility of the hindfoot, midfoot, and forefoot and possible passive correction of the deformity should be determined to distinguish rigid from flexible deformities. A thorough understanding of the pathomechanics of flat foot deformity allow for careful clinical assessment. Although the etiologies are numerous in the pediatric population, the progression of deformity over time is comparable to adult-acquired flat foot deformities. With progressive loss of the medial longitudinal arch and its supporting structures (ie, spring ligament, plantar aponeurosis, deltoid ligament, talocalcaneal ligament, and medial calcaneocuboid ligament), plantar flexion of the talar head occurs, with relaxation of the talonavicular capsule and midfoot abduction. This change progresses to the hindfoot, leading to valgus deformity and lateralization of the Achilles complex, as well as causing a compensatory forefoot supination in order to allow for a plantigrade foot position. The foot must be manipulated to assess the correction of hindfoot valgus as well as adduction of the navicular back over the uncovered talar head. It is important to note during the examination what happens to the forefoot when the heel is reduced to a neutral position, as additional procedures may be indicated to correct forefoot supination. Strength should be determined both manually and with testing of bilateral and single stance heel rise. With standing, the resting alignment of the heel should be visualized and correction into slight varus should be determined with heel rise. A "too-many-toes" sign should be assessed to indicate an increased midfoot abduction deformity (**Fig. 1**). Flexibility and correction of deformity can similarly be assessed by single heel rise testing or the Jack test, demonstrated by appearance of the medial arch with extension of the hallux. Gait should be analyzed both barefoot and with shoe wear. The shoes themselves should be analyzed for atypical wear pattern. The normal pattern regarding the heel is lateral wear. Patients with Achilles contractures often demonstrate little if any heel wear, with increased toe wear from increased forefoot loading. A pronation deformity may reveal increased wear of the medial counter and heel. Finally, a complete sensory and vascular examination should be performed.

RADIOLOGY

In most cases, routine radiographs for the patient presenting with asymptomatic flat foot is not required. However, various pathologies can lead to the development of

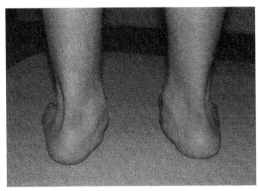

Fig. 1. Hindfoot valgus, medial plantar subluxation of the talar head, and a "too-many-toes" sign.

flat foot which, although it may be radiographically identifiable, may not yet become symptomatic to the patient, therefore radiographic examination is prudent. Weight-bearing anteroposterior (AP), lateral, and oblique views of the foot should be obtained. The authors also recommend weight-bearing views of the ankle joint to determine more proximal deformity and possible instability. To evaluate for accessory navicular, an internal rotation oblique view should be obtained. A calcaneonavicular coalition is best seen on the external rotation 45° oblique view. Even in the absence of history of trauma or growth plate injury, children with open physis with an orthopedic deformity should be evaluated radiographically for occult physeal pathology. The astute clinician should be careful not to miss rare cases where ankle deformity may be primarily driving the flat foot deformity. A multitude of radiographic measurements have been described for the evaluation of flat foot, but the most commonly used is the talar-first metatarsal angle or Meary angle: the angle subtended by a line drawn through the long axis of the talus and navicular in relation to the first metatarsal axis. A flat foot is associated with a negative Meary angle or one that is apex plantar (**Fig. 2**). Another important radiographic evaluation in the diagnosis and treatment of flat foot deformity includes the concept of talonavicular coverage (**Fig. 3**). When surgical management is indicated, the amount of talonavicular coverage can often dictate the choice of corrective procedures. Sangeorzan and colleagues[6] described radiographic assessment of flat foot deformity and correction of these radiographic parameters after lateral column lengthening. On the lateral foot view they described the lateral talocalcaneal angle, talometatarsal angle, and calcaneal length. On the AP foot view they

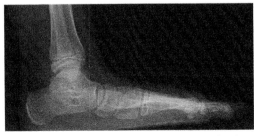

Fig. 2. Lateral radiograph showing typical deformity seen with flat foot and a flattening of the talar-first metatarsal angle.

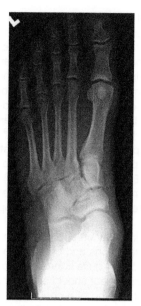

Fig. 3. Anteroposterior radiograph showing significant talonavicular uncoverage and abduction of the forefoot.

described the talometatarsal angle and the talonavicular coverage angle. The authors find the talonavicular coverage angle a very important determinant of correction and indicator of the extent of midfoot abduction. This angle is based on angular measurements obtained from the relationship of the center of the talus to the center of the navicular on the AP foot radiograph. In the Sangeorzan study there was an improvement of 26° in the alignment of these 2 articular surfaces after Evans calcaneal lengthening with insertion of a 1-cm allograft block.

More advanced imaging modalities such as computed tomography (CT), magnetic resonance imaging (MRI), and bone scan are not commonly indicated for the pain-free flexible flat foot, although special considerations apply. Considerable cost, burden to the patient, and possible poor patient tolerance should be considered when ordering further diagnostic studies. However, when specific or uncommon causes of flat foot deformity such as coalition or tumor are considered, CT scan and/or MRI may be illustrative. Often patients with coalition may not exhibit a classic "C" sign, talar beaking, or osseous bridging, and additional imaging studies are required to make the diagnosis.

TREATMENT: NONSURGICAL MANAGEMENT

Education and reassurance is the mainstay for treatment of the pain-free flexible flat foot. Patients and their parents alike should be counseled regarding the facts that the flat foot deformity may resolve with maturation (depending on the age of the patient and any underlying conditions) and that there exists no evidence that this deformity will lead to a painful condition in adulthood. Despite adequate education, patients and parents will seek some type of treatment with orthotic arch supports. However, there is no evidence to substantiate the assumption that orthoses will correct deformity or prevent future symptoms. Basmajian and Stecko[7] performed an electromyographic study of 20 adults, and concluded that the structure of the arch is dependent on the ligamentous and bony architecture and that the lower extremity muscles only play a significant role in maintenance of the arch with excessive loading. Studies have shown that although orthotic supports may aid in the correction of soft tissue deformities, the underlying bony architecture is unchanged. Bleck and Berninz[8] studied the effects of the Thomas heel in an over-the-counter insert and molded foot orthosis in a limited number of children, and found no radiographic improvement in flat foot deformity compared with the bare foot. The strongest support against the routine use of orthotics came from Wenger and colleagues[9] of the Texas Scottish Rite Hospital. These investigators performed a prospective study that compared a control group, a corrective shoe group, a Helfet heel cup group, and a custom-made plastic insert (University of California Biomechanics Laboratory) group. With a 3-year minimal follow-up, they concluded by radiographic and clinical examination that there was no statistical improvement or difference in the treated groups compared with the control group.

Orthotic supports and bracing may be appropriate for children who are symptomatic, although shoe wear modifications and other inexpensive modalities such as an off-the-shelf medial arch support are quite appropriate for initial management. Custom molded orthotics or custom shoe wear should only be reserved for those that fail the aforementioned modalities. Stretching of a contracted Achilles tendon and physical therapy may offer symptomatic benefit. The judicious use of nonsteroidal anti-inflammatories and other nonnarcotic pain medications is a useful adjunct.

TREATMENT: SURGICAL MANAGEMENT

The difficulty in management lies in the patient with a significant flat foot with some but minimal symptoms clearly attributable to the deformity. Although one should not be swayed into operative treatment based on the desires of the parents to have a child with a straight foot, difficulty lies in the unknown natural history, as stated previously. Although physiologic flat foot may resolve, the authors' experience has been that greater deformities do not. However, the inability to predict future symptomatology makes for a difficult decision on the part of the clinician. There is clearly a feel to the decision making in these cases, in essence the application of the "art" of medicine. Unfortunately, these difficult management decisions cannot be guided by radiographic parameters or more comfortably objective means. In the evaluation of these difficult cases the authors often ask, does form follow function or does function follow form? In the case of significant flat foot deformity in the pediatric population, the authors' experience has been that function follows form. Once the foot is better aligned, these patients have been found to have less likelihood of adult foot and ankle symptoms.

Surgical intervention can be categorized generally into soft tissue versus bone procedures, but often involves a combination of the two. Soft tissue procedures usually involve the Achilles tendon, posterior tibialis tendon, and peroneal tendons. The Achilles tendon can be lengthened for Achilles contractures. Depending on the area of contracture, a gastrocnemius recession or tendo-Achilles lengthening can be performed. Several procedures have been described that aim to alter the insertion of the posterior tibialis tendon. For example, Coleman and colleagues[10] reported 95% good to excellent results using the Durham procedure on 33 feet in 17 children. This procedure involves transfer or the posterior tibialis tendon along with elevation of a capsular and ligamentous flap to better tension the tendon and correct for the talonavicular coverage.

Bony procedures include the Kidner procedure for accessory navicular, coalition resection, arthroereisis, and various fusions and osteotomies. The choice of procedure is dependent on the underlying pathology as associated pathologic joints and the amount of correction required. There exists controversy as to the most appropriate intervention, as there are many satisfactory surgical options from which the surgeon can choose from. Particular care must be taken with the pediatric population due the presence of open physis and remaining growth potential. However, overall the exact principles that apply to adults apply to children as well. Choosing the correct procedure is a function of not only understanding the severity of deformity and flexibility of the hindfoot and forefoot, but is a function of surgeon comfort and skill. As the aforementioned procedures are discussed elsewhere in this issue, this discussion focuses on the use of the medial calcaneal translational osteotomy, the lateral column lengthening, medial cuneiform osteotomy, and calcaneal stop procedures.

The focus of this discussion is to highlight the use of osteotomies to correct deformity, that is, the medial translational and the lateral column calcaneal osteotomy as well as the opening wedge cuneiform osteotomy. In the authors' treatment algorithm this decision is driven by the presence of abduction of the midfoot which, if present, necessitates a lateral column calcaneal lengthening osteotomy. If, following the lengthening, heel valgus persists, then one can use an arthroereisis (discussed in another article in this issue), a medial translational calcaneal osteotomy, or a calcaneal stop procedure. If, following the lateral column lengthening, there is fixed forefoot supination, a medial cuneiform osteotomy must be performed.

Surgical management of the painful flexible flat foot in the pediatric population is indicated for patients with pain and dysfunction. Not all patients, in particular in the pediatric population, will present with classic symptoms such as medial foot pain, lateral impingement, or a history of significant disability. In fact there is a broad range of symptomatology with which children often present, and the astute clinician should elicit a history of shoe problems, difficulty running or keeping up with peers, and nonspecific aches in the legs, as well as the more typical medial arch discomfort and lateral symptoms from impingement.

Medial Calcaneal Translational Osteotomy

The initial concept of mechanically altering the axis or position of the calcaneus to better normalize deformity was first described by Gleich in 1893.[11] However, it was Koutsogiannis who first recognized that sliding the calcaneus medially improves outcomes in flexible pes planus.[12] The medial calcaneal translational osteotomy is a valuable intervention whenever hindfoot valgus exists and when the medial foot needs to be supported. Successful correction of flat foot deformity involves restoring the heel to normal alignment, as procedures that focus only on the forefoot and neglect the hindfoot valgus will usually fail. The medial translation has several benefits aside from correcting the position of the bony hindfoot. Medial translation can help normalize contact pressures if valgus deformity is seen at the ankle. In addition, it shifts the weight-bearing axis of the heel under the long axis of the tibia. This procedure also medializes the Achilles insertion in relation to the subtalar joint, increasing its biomechanical function but on the subtalar joint. Several researchers, including Nyska and colleagues[13] and Sung and colleagues,[14] have shown that medial calcaneal translational osteotomy can have the additional effects of preventing flat foot deformity by eliminating the negative deforming effects of Achilles tendon and improving the outcome of flexor digitorum longus transfer, respectively. In other words, the gastrocnemius acts positively on the fulcrum of the subtalar joint following the calcaneus osteotomy.

An incision is made along the lateral hindfoot approximately 2 fingerbreadths below the tip of the lateral malleolus in line with the peroneal tendons. As the incision is deepened into subcutaneous tissue, the sural nerve and lesser saphenous vein should be identified and carefully protected. Once retractors are placed, deeper dissection can be performed safely. The periosteum overlying the planned osteotomy is incised and the calcaneus exposed. After subperiosteal dissection, 2 curved retractors are placed both dorsally and plantar around the tuberosity. The osteotomy cut is made perpendicular to the axis of the tuberosity at a 45° angle with respect to the calcaneal pitch or approximately in line with the axis of the subtalar joint. The osteotomy cut is made with a sagittal saw, with care taken as the medial cortex is breached to protect the medial neurovascular and tendinous structures. Next, a smooth laminar spreader is placed and the medial periosteum is separated sharply. The medial translation is performed with translation of approximately 10 to 12 mm, taking care not to translate superiorly or inferiorly. The translation is initially stabilized with 1 or 2 guide wires inserted from the posterior heel across the osteotomy site, which are checked under fluoroscopy for adequate translation of the osteotomy and avoidance of the subtalar joint. Choice of fixation is dependent on the age of the patient and whether the calcaneal physis is open or closed. If closed or reaching skeletal maturity, the construct can be stabilized with one 6.5-mm cannulated screw. If skeletally immature with significant growth remaining, the osteotomy can be stabilized with smooth pin fixation. The wound is thoroughly irrigated and closed in layered fashion. Once the hindfoot is corrected, attention is turned to the forefoot. Depending on the amount of deformity, often additional procedures are now required.

Lateral Column Lengthening (Evans Procedure)

Often the deformity is such that lateral column lengthening is required to correct residual forefoot abduction and talonavicular coverage. Calcaneal cuboid arthrodesis is an alternative to lengthening osteotomy in the adult population with significant forefoot abduction, arthritis, and/or greater than 40% talonavicular uncoverage. However, in the pediatric population with an open physis and growth potential, lengthening is the preferred procedure. Sangeorzan and colleagues[6] performed a cadaveric study in 1993 using the Evans procedure and found significant improvements in talonavicular coverage, talometatarsal angle, and calcaneal pitch angle.

The incision is made along the lateral foot over the dorsal surface of the peroneal tendons extending from the tip of the lateral malleolus to the calcaneocuboid joint. The incision should be slightly more dorsal then straight lateral, as the rest of the procedure is facilitated by exposing the calcaneal neck from a dorsal lateral approach versus a straight lateral approach. Care must be taken to identify and protect the sural nerve. Deeper dissection is performed and the peroneal tendons are retracted inferiorly. The periosteum on the neck of the calcaneus is sharply incised and elevated dorsally so that the anterior aspect of the subtalar joint is completely visualized.

Next, the neck of the calcaneus is cut with a sagittal saw perpendicular to the long axis of the calcaneus and approximately 10 mm proximal to the calcaneocuboid joint (**Fig. 4**). The osteotomy is carried medially between the middle and anterior calcaneal facets, and it is useful to verify the position of the osteotomy with a k-wire under fluoroscopy first (**Fig. 5**). This method is in contradistinction to the osteotomy as described by Hintermann and colleagues,[15] which crosses the calcaneus between the posterior and middle calcaneal facet. The authors recognize that a precise osteotomy between the middle and anterior calcaneal facets may be difficult due to inadequate visualization during the procedure, and possible normal variations not only in facet position but also congenital singular and combined middle/anterior facet. However, the ability to

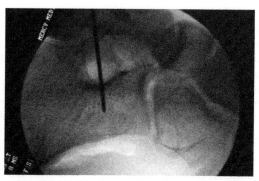

Fig. 4. Intraoperative fluoroscopy showing site for planned osteotomy.

correct midfoot abduction is increased by a lengthening in closer proximity to the calcaneal cuboid joint. In other words, an osteotomy more distal and in closer proximity to the apex of deformity allows for a more powerful correction of the abduction deformity, permitting increased adduction of the midfoot and thus increasing talar coverage by the navicular. Furthermore, it is essential to recognize that when a laminar spreader is inserted into the calcaneus for lengthening, the forefoot adducts and rotates over the navicular, but the calcaneal tuberosity also shifts slightly posteriorly. As the tuberosity moves posteriorly, there will be impingement against the posterior facet and the osteotomy will fail due to postoperative pain in the sinus tarsi. Postoperative pain in the sinus tarsi associated with normal alignment usually implies some impingement of the neck of the calcaneus against the posterior facet.

Both cortices should be penetrated and manually loosened with an osteotome. The medial cortex can be penetrated to obtain adequate hinging and lengthening of the

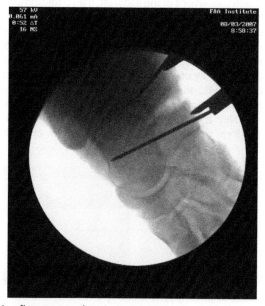

Fig. 5. Intraoperative fluoroscopy showing osteotomy.

lateral column. Next, a smooth laminar spreader is inserted into the osteotomy site onto the thicker cortical bone and gently expanded while the foot is examined both clinically and under fluoroscopy. Correction of forefoot abduction and talonavicular coverage is carefully assessed at this time. If correction is adequate the amount of distraction at the osteotomy site is measured (usually about 10 mm), and an appropriately sized and shaped allograft is fashioned usually from iliac crest or femoral head allograft (**Figs. 6** and **7**). The other alternative for distraction of the osteotomy is to use a custom-designed plate that has a small wedge to maintain the osteotomy distracted; it is a 4-hole locking plate, which can be augmented in the osteotomy site with a small amount of cancellous bone (DePuy, Warsaw, IN, USA). Insertion of a graft can be difficult because it can be limited by the position of the laminar spreader, so that a pin distractor may be more useful, as it does not get in the way of the graft. Once the graft is tamped into place, position and foot alignment should be rechecked under fluoroscopy. Care must be taken to not translate the graft dorsally, as this will cause abutment against the anterior aspect of the subtalar joint and painful impingement, and any anterior impingement is removed with a saw or rongeur.

There are several pitfalls to this procedure that the surgeon should be aware of. Intraoperatively the sural nerve must be carefully identified and retracted. Similarly, the peroneal tendons are at risk and need to be protected from inadvertent laceration. The osteotomy must be carefully planned, as fracture of the distal calcaneus can occur if the osteotomy is made too close the calcaneal cuboid joint. One must try to avoid dorsal subluxation of the distal segment of the neck of the calcaneus on the cuboid when distracting. If this occurs, a temporary k-wire can be inserted across the calcaneocuboid joint to hold it in place; alternatively distract the calcaneus a little less. Nonunion and calcaneal cuboid arthritis are extremely rare following the osteotomy in the child. A more common complication, however, is unrecognized dorsal displacement of the distal segment against the subtalar joint. With dorsal translation of the distal calcaneus, impingement of the anterior calcaneus can occur, resulting in pain and a less than optimal outcome; this can occur for several reasons, including the osteotomy itself and placement of the allograft. If an osteotomy is made incorrectly and not perpendicular to the long axis of the calcaneus, this can result in translation of the distal fragment. Given the original deformity and need for correction of forefoot supination, the distal segment is often inadvertently displaced dorsally due to the intact capsular and ligamentous attachments between the distal calcaneus and cuboid. Similarly, this deformity can be caused or exacerbated by improper fashioning of the allograft. If a trapezoidal graft is fashioned with a smaller relative length dorsally, this may cause dorsal translation of the distal fragment. Although some investigators describe inherent stability and forgo internal fixation, the authors have found that internal fixation in the form of a k-wire, a cannulated screw, or a 4-hole custom plate

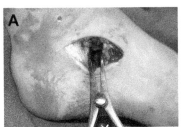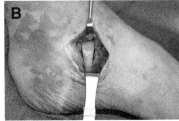

Fig. 6. (*A, B*) Intraoperative photographs showing osteotomy site distracted by a laminar spreader and placement of a fashioned femoral head allograft.

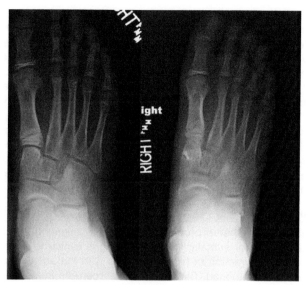

Fig. 7. Anteroposterior view of the foot before and after lateral column lengthening, showing improvement in talonavicular coverage.

is the most reliable way of ensuring a stable construct and avoiding dorsal displacement of the distal segment. Kimball and colleagues[16] demonstrated that a cervical H-plate afforded higher stiffness and load to failure compared with 2 crossed 3.5-mm cortical lag screws in a cadaver model assessing fixation of calcaneocuboid distraction arthrodesis.

Medial Cuneiform Osteotomy

Once the lateral column lengthening has been performed, the forefoot should be carefully examined clinically for a fixed supination deformity, and if residual forefoot supination is present, a medial procedure is required to plantarflex the first ray. One cannot assume that the peroneus longus will be strong enough in the future to pull the first metatarsal into equinus, correcting the forefoot supination. The best choice for correction of this deformity in the pediatric population is an opening wedge osteotomy of the medial cuneiform. Arthrodesis of the first tarsometatarsal can be used in the adult, but unless gross hypermobility is present it is not be the best option in the child. Similarly, a first metatarsal osteotomy is contraindicated due to open physis. This procedure was first described by Cotton to restore the "triangle of support of the static foot."[17] As an adjunct procedure, it helps with correction of forefoot supination and improves the declination of the first ray, improving medial forefoot weight bearing.

An incision is made over the dorsal aspect of the medial midfoot immediately medial to the extensor hallucis longus tendon and lateral to the anterior tibial tendon. Care must be taken to identify and protect superficial cutaneous branches of the superficial peroneal nerve, as well as to avoid the deep peroneal nerve and dorsal pedal artery during deeper dissection. The medial cuneiform is exposed with subperiosteal dissection and a guide pin is inserted from dorsal to plantar, aiming slightly proximal. The positioning is checked under fluoroscopy to ensure adequate placement and that the pin is located centrally in the cuneiform. A saw cut is next made on either side of the guide pin with care not to penetrate the distal plantar cortex. The guide pin is removed and the osteotomy is opened using an osteotome. A laminar spreader is placed for distraction, and the correction is checked clinically and under fluoroscopy. Once adequate correction is noted, the amount of distraction at the osteotomy site is measured (usually 6 mm) and a trapezoidal or triangular graft (wider dorsally with apex plantar) is fashioned and inserted. Once the graft is tamped into place, position and foot alignment should be rechecked under fluoroscopy. Usually the press-fit graft is stable, but a fully threaded 4-mm cancellous screw can be placed from the dorsal surface at the level of the metatarsal cuneiform joint aiming proximally, or even a k-wire introduced percutaneously. Finally, any overlying graft that may cause impingement is carefully removed with a rongeur, and the wound is thoroughly irrigated and closed in layered fashion.

Correction of flat foot deformity after lateral column lengthening and medial cuneiform osteotomy is demonstrated in **Fig. 8.**

Calcaneal Stop Procedure

The goals of the calcaneal stop procedure of properly orienting the talus over the calcaneus and allowing for subtalar joint remodeling is similar to arthroereisis. This procedure allows for correction of hindfoot valgus with the advantages of maintenance of some subtalar motion. Similar to an arthroereisis implant, the calcaneal stop acts as an "internal orthotic device" and can be placed almost percutaneously, with minimal morbidity and recovery time. The calcaneal stop functions in a mechanical way as well as having a proprioceptive function. Whereas the indications for subtalar arthroereisis are broad, the indications for the calcaneal stop technique have not been determined. The calcaneal stop procedure may have an advantage over subtalar arthroereisis, as the blocking screw is not placed across the subtalar joint but instead into the calcaneus to prevent hindfoot eversion. Several studies have reported on complications following subtalar arthroereisis including granuloma formation, implant displacement, biomaterial failure, tissue staining, implant irritation, and sinus tarsi pain.[18–20] Theoretically the calcaneal stop procedure may reduce some of these complications. Roth and colleagues[21] reported using this technique for idiopathic flexible pes planovalgus deformity in children. From 1997 to 2003, 94 procedures were done on 48 children between the ages of 8 and 14 years. The Meary angle to determine the degree of collapse of the medial longitudinal arch was 170° or less, and the weight-bearing hindfoot was in valgus. The screw presumably achieves correction by stimulating the proprioceptive foot receptors, allowing active inversion of the foot. At 5 years' follow-up, no serious complications occurred. In every foot, heel valgus

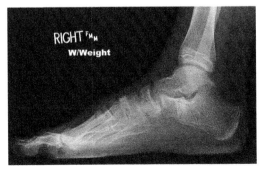

Fig. 8. Lateral radiograph before and after lateral column lengthening and medial cuneiform osteotomy, showing correction of flat foot deformity.

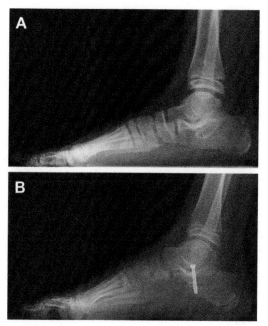

Fig. 9. Lateral radiograph before (*A*) and after (*B*) calcaneal stop procedure, showing improvement in flat foot deformity.

and the longitudinal arch of the foot were improved radiographically and clinically, without loss of function. Jerosch and colleagues described results using this technique in 21 flat feet in the pediatric population from 1999 to 2007.[22] These investigators noted significant improvement in heel valgus during rest and tiptoeing, significant improvement in dorsiflexion, and improvement in talonavicular angulation.

A 2-cm incision is made over the sinus tarsi. Care is taken to avoid the sural nerve and retractors are placed. Then under fluoroscopic guidance, a guide wire is placed vertically into the calcaneus from superior to inferior as the heel is held in a reduced position. This is overdrilled with a 3.2-mm drill, and a 6.5-mm cancellous screw of approximately 30 to 35 mm length is inserted such that the screw head impinges against the lateral aspect of the talus, preventing eversion at the subtalar joint. Positioning of the screw and maintenance of normal heel position is checked under fluoroscopy. Finally, the wound is thoroughly irrigated and closed in layered fashion (**Fig. 9**).

SUMMARY

The flexible flat foot is treated according to the location of the deformity, ie, hindfoot valgus, midfoot abduction, and forefoot supination. There is generally a contracture of the gastrocnemius requiring treatment, which is performed in conjunction with osteotomy of the calcaneus and cuneiform as required.

REFERENCES

1. Staheli LT, Chew DE, Corbett M. The longitudinal arch: a survey of eight hundred and eighty-two feet in normal children and adults. J Bone Joint Surg Am 1987;69:426–8.

2. Gould N, Moreland M, Alvarez R, et al. Development of the child's arch. Foot Ankle 1989;9:241.

3. Rao UB, Joseph B. The influence of footwear on the prevalence of flat foot: a survey of 2300 children. J Bone Joint Surg Br 1992;74:525–7 [see comments].

4. Sachithanandam V, Joseph B. The influence of footwear on the prevalence of flat foot: a survey of 1846 skeletally mature persons. J Bone Joint Surg Br 1995;77: 254–7.

5. Harris RI, Beath T. Army foot survey: an investigation of the foot ailments of Canadian soldiers. Ottowa Nat Res Council 1947;1:52.

6. Sangeorzan B, Mosca V, Hansen S. Effect of calcaneal lengthening on relationships among the hindfoot, midfoot, and forefoot. Foot Ankle 1993;14:136–41.

7. Basmajian JV, Stecko G. The role of muscles in arch support of the foot: an electromyographic study. J Bone Joint Surg Am 1963;45:1184–90.

8. Bleck EE, Berninz UJ. Conservative management of pes valgus with plantar flexed talus. Clin Orthop 1977;122:85–94.

9. Wenger DR, Mauldin D, Speck G, et al. Corrective shoes and inserts as treatment for flexible flat foot in infants and children. J Bone Joint Surg Am 1989;71:800–10 [see comments].

10. Coleman SS, Stelling FH III, Jarrett J. Pathomechanics and treatment of congenital vertical talus. Clin Orthop 1970;70:62–72.

11. Gleich A. Beitrag zur operative Plattfussbehandlung. Arch Klin Chir 1893;46: 358–62 [in German].

12. Koutsogiannis E. Treatment of mobile flat foot by displacement osteotomy of the calcaneus. J Bone Joint Surg Br 1971;53(1):96–100.

13. Nyska M, Parks BG, Chu IT, et al. The contribution of the medial calcaneal osteotomy to the correction of flatfoot deformities. Foot Ankle Int 2001;22(4):278–82.

14. Sung IH, Lee S, Otis JC, et al. Posterior tibial tendon force requirement in early heel rise after calcaneal osteotomies. Foot Ankle Int 2002;23(9):842–9.

15. Hintermann B, Valderrabano V, Kundert HP. Lengthening of the lateral column and reconstruction of the medial soft tissue for treatment of acquired flat foot deformity associated with insufficiency of the posterior tibial tendon. Foot Ankle Int 1999;20(10):622–9.

16. Kimball HL, Aronow MS, Sullivan RJ, et al. Biomechanical evaluation of calcaneocuboid distraction arthrodesis: a cadaver study of two different fixation methods. Foot Ankle Int 2000;21(10):845–8.

17. Cotton FJ. Foot statics and surgery. N Engl J Med 1936;214:353–62.

18. Carranza A, Gimeno V, Gomez JA, et al. Giannini's prosthesis in the treatment of juvenile flatfoot. J Foot Ankle Surg 2000;6:11–7.

19. Saxena A, Nguyen A. Preliminary radiographic findings and sizing implications on patients undergoing bioabsorbable subtalar arthroereisis. J Foot Ankle Surg 2007;46(3):175–80.

20. Miller SJ. The MBA subtalar joint implant in the adult flexible flat foot: preliminary data and experience. Reconstructive surgery foot and ankle update 98. Tucker (GA): The Podiatry Institute; 1998. p. 99–117.

21. Roth S, Sestan B, Tudor A, et al. Minimally invasive calcaneo-stop method for idiopathic flexible pes planovalgus in children. Foot Ankle Int 2007;28(9):991–5.

22. Jerosch J, Schunck J, Abdel-Aziz H. The stop screw technique-a simple and reliable method in treating flexible flatfoot in children. J Foot Ankle Surg 2009;15(4): 174–8.

Subtalar Arthroereisis in Pediatric Flatfoot Reconstruction

Pablo Fernández de Retana, MD[a],*, Fernándo Álvarez, MD[b],
Ramón Viladot, MD[c]

KEYWORDS

• Arthroereisis • Subtalar implant • Flatfoot • Subtalar joint
• Pes planovalgus • Pediatric flatfoot

Pediatric and juvenile flatfoot is a common problem in childhood, present in one in nine children.[1] The morphologic characteristics of this condition are heel valgus and flattening of the medial longitudinal arch. Other characteristics are usually observed, such as supination and abduction of the forefoot, tightening of the Achilles tendon, and hypertonia of the peroneal muscles. Most children with flatfoot will undergo spontaneous correction or become asymptomatic; those that are symptomatic require treatment.

Conservative treatment includes supportive footwear and physical therapy. Usually flatfoot is overtreated. The prevalence of flat feet with diagnostic criteria was 2.7% in a Spanish population of 4- to 13-year-old schoolchildren, with 14.2% of them were receiving orthopedic treatment.[2] Very little is known about the natural development of flatfoot, and failure to treat this condition could lead to persistent pain in the medial longitudinal arch, hallux valgus, degenerative arthritis, posterior tibial tendon dysfunction, metatarsalgia, and knee or low back pain.[3,4]

Surgery is rarely indicated in children with flatfeet. Surgical options are tendon transfers, tarsal arthrodeses, calcaneal osteotomies, and subtalar joint motion blocking procedures. The final decision is usually based on the clinical and radiographic assessment of the patient and surgeon preference. Flexible flatfoot should be treated preferably with extra-articular procedures and avoiding tendon transfers. In 1946, Chambers[5] was the first to introduce the idea of restricting subtalar joint motion

[a] Department of Orthopedic Surgery, Hospital San Rafael, Passeig Vall d'Hebron 107-117, 08035 Barcelona, Spain
[b] Head of Foot and Ankle Unit, Department of Orthopedic Surgery, Hospital San Rafael, Passeig Vall d'Hebron 107-117, 08035 Barcelona, Spain
[c] Clínica Tres Torres, Barcelona, Spain
* Corresponding author.
E-mail address: pfernan@hsrafael.com

Foot Ankle Clin N Am 15 (2010) 323–335
doi:10.1016/j.fcl.2010.01.001
1083-7515/10/$ – see front matter © 2010 Elsevier Inc. All rights reserved.

foot.theclinics.com

with an autologous bone block filling the sinus tarsi. In 1952, Grice[6] observed that extra-articular subtalar arthrodesis with cortical graft for flatfoot deformity in children was associated with several problems, such as development of degenerative arthritis in adjacent joints and inability of the hindfoot to adapt to uneven surfaces. Haraldsson[7] and Lelievre[8] pointed out it was most important to block the sinus tarsi restricting subtalar motion while avoiding arthrodesis. Since then, the term *arthroereisis* is used to describe the limitation of subtalar motion.[8]

Shortening of the gastrocnemius or the Achilles tendon is very common in flatfoot, and often these structures need to be lengthened. Osteoperiosteal flap of the posterior tibial tendon has been advised to increase the strength of this muscle. In the past, this procedure was recommended in addition to arthroereisis, whereas now arthroereisis is performed without the osteoperiosteal flap.

SUBTALAR ARTHROEREISIS WITH SINUS TARSI IMPLANT

Arthroereisis has been used predominantly in recent years to treat flatfeet in the pediatric population.[9,10] Many arthroereisis procedures have been described to limit subtalar joint motion and improve position. In 1970, Lelievre[8] introduced the term *lateral arthroereisis* using a temporary staple across the subtalar joint. In 1977, Subotnick[11] first described a sinus tarsi implant using a block of silicone elastamer. Smith and Millar[3] used a polyethylene screw in sinus tarsi (STA-peg, Dow Corning Wright Corporation, Arlington, TN, USA) and reported a 96% success rate. Vedantam and colleagues[12] used the STA-peg in 78 patients, most of whom had neurologic problems, and reported satisfactory results in 96%. Although no implant degradation was encountered, they did not recommend the implant in more active children.

Viladot[4] reported the use of a silicon implant with a cup shape, obtaining 99% good results in 234 patients. Carranza-Bencano and colleagues[13] obtained 90% good and excellent results in 77 feet with Viladot's silicon implant. Using Viladot's device, Black and colleagues[14] were unable to obtain consistent improvements radiologically, and 73% of patients reported that their feet were significantly painful.

Currently, silicon implants are not usually used and have been replaced with tronco-conical implants, such as Kalix (Newdeal, Saint Priest, France) and MBA (Kinetikos Medical, Inc, Carlsbad, CA, USA). Zaret and Myerson[9] reported 23 children who had flexible flatfoot treated with MBA implants. They reported postoperative sinus tarsi pain in 18% of patients that improved with rest and corticosteroid injection. Two children required implant removal at a mean of 9 months after surgery. Subtalar joint range of motion increased after implant removal. They also observed an interesting phenomenon: removal of the implant was not associated with a reversal of the foot structure.

Giannini[15] developed an expanding and bioabsorbable implant material. He reported 94% good results in 50 cases using nonreabsorbable material and 20 cases with bioabsorbable. He observed no difference in long-term follow-up between nonreabsorbable and bioabsorbable materials. Bioabsorbable implants have the advantage of a low rate of intolerance, which helps avoid a second procedure for removal.

The "calcaneo-stop" is a technique for limiting motion in the subtalar joint through the insertion of a screw into the calcaneus. Álvarez[16] was the first to describe this procedure using a cancellous screw (**Fig. 1**). The entry point was located in the sinus tarsi. The head of the screw limits talus motion and prevents talus displacement downward. In 475 patients with an average follow-up ranging from 12 to 112 months, Magnan and colleagues[17] reported 83% good results. Nogarin[18] described the anterograde calcaneus-stop with a cancellous screw inserted into the talus. Recently, Roth

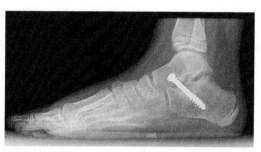

Fig. 1. Recaredo's procedure.

and colleagues[19] reported 94 feet operated in 48 children using a temporary cancellous screw placed percutaneously into the talus. At 5 years follow-up, 91.5% had excellent results.

Vogler[20] classified sinus tarsi implants into three types based on their biomechanical properties: self-locking wedge, axis-altering implant, and impact-blocking device. Most sinus tarsi implants are self-locking wedge. All sinus tarsi devices restrict hindfoot valgus, and the calcaneus is vertically orientated beneath the ankle joint.[10] The talus is dorsiflexed and externally deviated. Talonavicular subluxation and forefoot abduction are corrected.

INDICATIONS FOR SUBTALAR ARTHROEREISIS IN CHILDREN

Supportive insoles with a medial longitudinal arch are recommended in children who have painful flatfoot. Surgery is indicated for symptomatic flatfoot, which persists despite prolonged nonsurgical treatment. Surgical options are lateral column lengthening and sinus tarsi implant. Both operations need a flexible foot to correct malposition. If a rigid deformity of the foot is present (eg, tarsal coalitions or spastic disorders), additional procedures must be associated.

Calcaneal lengthening is widely accepted in the United States, whereas sinus tarsi implants have been used for many years in European countries. The advantages of arthroereisis over osteotomies are that it is easy to perform, less immobilization is required, and it has no associated risk for nonunion. However, its disadvantages include a high percentage of implant intolerance and limitation of subtalar motion. No controlled trials are comparing these techniques and the level of scientific evidence is low. Practitioners using both techniques agree that a low percentage of children who have flexible flatfoot require surgery.[15,21]

Pediatric flatfoot can have different origins, including flexible flatfoot, cerebral palsy, myelomeningocele, tarsal coalitions, and rheumatic diseases. Not every child's flatfoot needs surgical treatment and, when surgery is necessary, not all cases require subtalar arthroereisis. The main indications of subtalar arthroereisis in children are discussed in the following sections.

Flexible Flatfoot

Flexible flatfoot is a very common disorder in children. It rarely needs surgical treatment because patients are usually completely asymptomatic and most of these feet correct spontaneously with growth. However, in a small group of these patients (<3%), the feet do not correct and are symptomatic. Symptoms are pain (usually on the medial side of the foot), fatigue, difficulty playing sports or walking on uneven surfaces, and cramps. Surgery is indicated in these patients if, in addition to symptoms, the child demonstrates most of the following inclusion criteria: severe flat-foot without clinical and radiologic improvement after at least 2 years of conservative treatment; hindfoot valgus greater than 10°; shortness of the Achilles tendon; Viladot footprint type II, III, or IV[4]; talo-first metatarsal (Meary's) angle smaller that 170°; Moreau-Costa-Bartani angle greater than 130°, or Kite angle greater than 25°.

The age of the patient is an important factor and is of wide concern.[3,15] The authors recommend surgery between 8 and 12 years. Before 8 years, many children may experience spontaneous correction. The authors also prefer not to operate on patients older than 12 years of age because one goal of arthroereisis is to relocate the talus properly over the calcaneus to allow remodeling of these bones and the subtalar joint during the rest of the growing period, which they believe requires at least 2 years. The sinus tarsi implant acts as a splint restoring the normal foot architecture. Bone growth will develop in the right way. After 12 years of age, there is not enough time for remodeling hindfoot bones and ligaments. Although many children have flexible flatfeet, very few meet the inclusion criteria, and therefore surgery is unusual for childhood flexible flatfoot.

Flatfoot Associated to Navicular Bone Disorders

It is not unusual for childhood flatfoot to be related to an accessory or a prominent navicular. In these cases, the tibialis posterior tendon has an abnormal distal insertion, which may cause a functional insufficiency of this tendon. If the foot is symptomatic, subtalar arthroereisis must be associated with partial removal of the navicular as described by Kidner,[22] or a suture between both tibialis tendons.

Flatfoot Associated With Tarsal Coalition

Talocalcaneal and calcaneonavicular coalitions can cause flatfoot. Usually this condition is asymptomatic until the age of 10 to 12 years, when the foot becomes painful, the hindfoot is stiff, and a painful contracture of the peroneal tendons occurs. When surgery is needed, removal of the coalition is indicated together with subtalar arthroereisis. If more than one third of the subtalar joint is affected, subtalar arthrodesis is probably a better option.

Flatfoot Secondary to Clubfoot Overcorrection

Flatfeet that are secondary to clubfoot overcorrection are difficult to correct because they are stiff from previous treatments. However, in some cases the foot is still flexible and subtalar arthroereisis may be indicated. Additional surgical procedures are often necessary to correct forefoot deformities (hallux flexus is frequent in overcorrected clubfeet).

Spastic Paralytic Flatfoot

Children who have cerebral palsy often develop severe planovalgus feet with Achilles and peroneal tendons contracture. Arthrodesis or tendon transfers are accepted treatments. When the foot is not very rigid, subtalar arthroereisis can be an alternative to arthrodesis.[23]

Subtalar arthroereisis should only be indicated in patients who have severe symptomatic flatfoot that has not improved with orthotic treatment and who fulfill the inclusion criteria for flexible flat foot.

COMPLICATIONS

Complications may be divided into general and implant-specific.[10] General complications include persistent sinus tarsi pain, malposition, overcorrection, undercorrection, wrong implant size, and loss of position.[10] The most common complication is intolerance of the implant because of pain. Black and colleagues[14] reported 73% painful feet using Viladot's initial design, requiring implant removal in 36% of their patients with little resolution of the symptoms. This initial design by Viladot is no longer used. Gutiérrez and Herrera[24] reported that 7.5% of implant removals involved the Giannini non-reabsorbable implant. Overcorrection is a cause of pain in sinus tarsi and implant removal has been recommended with good results (**Fig. 2**).[12]

Implant-specific complications are related to the properties of each implant, and include debris from wear, foreign body reaction, implant degradation, and implant fracture.[10] For Roth and colleagues,[19] 12% of complications were related to the calcaneo-stop technique, and all were associated with the screws (9 screw breakages and 2 incorrectly positioned screws). Giannini[15] reported two complications involving implant degradation (4.8%) in his series with a bioreabsorbable implant. Small fragments migrated under the skin, causing local irritation.

Arthritis, synovitis, implant fracture, and implant loosening have been reported with the STA-peg implant.[3] Case reports have shown intraosseous cysts within the talus,[25] osteonecrosis of the talus,[26] peroneal muscle spasms, and small fracture of the calcaneus.[27]

Gutiérrez and Herrera[24] reported temporary postoperative supination in 27% of cases. This condition resolved spontaneously in all feet, but resolution of symptoms took 1 month in 35%, 3 months in 41%, and 4 months in 24% of cases.

SURGICAL TECHNIQUE

The authors usually perform foot surgery under general anesthesia in children. The patient is placed in a supine position with a pillow under the ipsilateral buttock to avoid excessive external rotation of the foot and facilitate approach to the sinus tarsi. A

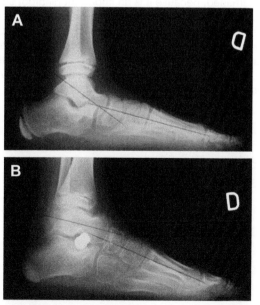

Fig. 2. Preoperative (*A*) and postoperative (*B*) lateral radiographs showing overcorrection after subtalar arthroereisis.

pneumatic tourniquet is applied at the thigh and the surgical field is prepared leaving the leg exposed.

In most cases, the first step of the operation is the lengthening of the Achilles tendon. To evaluate if this tendon is retracted, the authors hold the foot with the hindfoot in neutral position and the knee completely extended. Then we passively dorsiflex the foot. If we cannot achieve 10° of dorsiflexion we consider that the Achilles tendon is retracted and needs to be lengthened, which will help in correcting valgus of the calcaneus and implanting the endorthesis. They recommend percutaneous lengthening. Two 5-mm incisions are performed on the lateral border of the tendon (at 2 and 6 cm from its insertion in the calcaneus) and one 5-mm incision on the medial border (at 4 cm from the insertion). Through each incision, the tendon is divided transversely approximately half of its width. The foot is dorsiflexed so that the tendon is lengthened until approximately 15° of dorsiflexion is obtained while the knee is extended.

If an accessory or prominent navicular bone must be removed, the procedure is performed as described by Kidner.[22] A 3-cm longitudinal skin incision is performed at the medial side of the foot, over the navicular tuberosity. The tibialis posterior tendon is split and partially detached from the navicular bone. The bony prominence or accessory bone is removed and the tendon sutured. Subcutaneous tissue and skin are also sutured.

A slightly curved 2-cm skin incision is made on the lateral side of the hindfoot centered over the sinus tarsi, just anterior and plantar to the tip of the lateral malleolus. Care must be taken not to damage the peroneal tendons, saphenous nerve, and intermediate dorsal cutaneous nerve (a branch of the superficial peroneal nerve). Direct approach to the sinus tarsi is obtained. The sinus tarsi is debrided to remove its contents (fatty tissue with abundant nerve endings) (**Fig. 3**). This step is important to eliminate the irritative stimuli of the endorthesis in the sinus, which could originate the contracture of the peroneal tendons. The powerful interosseous talocalcaneal ligament must not be damaged, because it is an important hindfoot stabilizer.

The next step consists of restoration of the foot arch and correction of calcaneus valgus deviation. This is achieved using a blunt lever introduced through the sinus tarsi and under the neck of the talus. The correcting procedure is then performed, with the lever pushed in distal direction so that the hindfoot is supinated at the same time the assistant pronates the forefoot. The aim of this procedure is to move the head of the talus upwards, backward, and outwards, so that it is repositioned in its physiologic

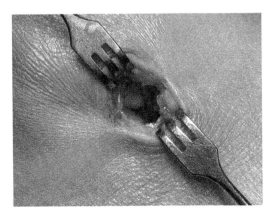

Fig. 3. Sinus tarsi is emptied.

position and hindfoot pronation is corrected. One must note that in flatfoot, the talus has slipped forward, downward, and inward.

To conserve the correction obtained, an endorthesis is inserted in the sinus tarsi. First, the trial implants (with increasing diameters) are inserted until the appropriate implant size is determined. The authors choose the smallest implant that corrects the deformity and remains stable in the sinus tarsi while moving the subtalar joint. It is advisable to check the correct position of the trial implant with fluoroscopy. Then, the definitive endorthesis is implanted, which is the same size as the trial implant (**Fig. 4**).

Closure of the wound is performed in a routine fashion and a below-knee compression cast is applied. The whole procedure takes 20 to 30 minutes.

If necessary, additional procedures can be associated, such as removal of accessory navicular bone, removal of tarsal coalition, and peroneal tendons lengthening.

Sutures are removed 10 to 12 days postoperatively and a below knee walking cast is applied. This cast is removed 6 weeks after surgery and the patient is advised to wear rigid orthopedic insoles for 1 year to support the correction. Weight-bearing is allowed when the skin has healed.

Endorthesis

Since 1998, the authors have been using the Kalix endorthesis (Newdeal SA, Vienne, France) for child and adult flatfoot surgical treatment (**Fig. 5**). This implant consists of a metal cone trunk introduced into another polyethylene cone trunk that expands. It is manufactured with the biocompatible materials titanium and high-density polyethylene. Its conical shape fits well into the sinus tarsi, and the lateral fins prevent the implant from moving out of the sinus tarsi. It can be visualized radiographically because of its metallic component.

RESULTS OF TREATMENT

In 2006, the authors performed a descriptive retrospective study of children who had flatfoot treated with subtalar arthroereisis between 1998 and 2005 in their institution, Hospital San Rafael in Barcelona, Spain. The total number of feet operated was 116 in 68 patients. Etiology of the deformity showed flexible flatfoot in 97 feet; tarsal coalition in 10 feet; spastic flatfoot in 3 feet; Down's syndrome in 2 feet; clubfoot overcorrection in 2 feet; and juvenile arthritis in 2 feet. To have a homogeneous sample, the study only included patients who had flexible flatfoot (56 patients and 97 feet).

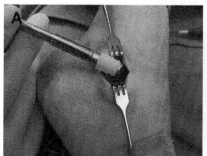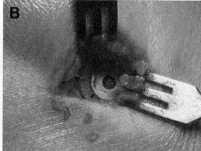

Fig. 4. (*A*) Endorthesis mounted on its handle and ready to be implanted. (*B*) Endorthesis implanted in sinus tarsi.

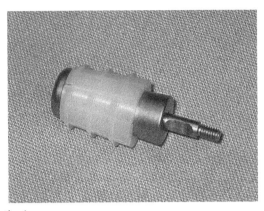

Fig. 5. Kalix endorthesis.

The average age at surgery was 10.5 years (range, 7–14 years), and the mean follow-up was 4.5 years (range, 1.1–8.0 years). The patients consisted of 34 boys (60.1%) and 22 girls (39.9%), and side distribution was 50 right feet (51.5%) and 47 left (48.5%).

All 97 feet underwent subtalar arthroereisis with Kalix endorthesis and the Achilles tendon was lengthened in 85 feet (87.6%).

The study included clinical and radiologic evaluation, and the American Orthopaedic Foot & Ankle Society (AOFAS) scale was used. The footprint evolution was also evaluated. The radiological study consisted of weight-bearing anteroposterior and lateral views of both feet. In the anterior-posterior view, the angle between the main axes of the talus and calcaneus (Kite angle, which should be between 15° and 25°) was measured. In the lateral view, the Moreau-Costa-Bartani angle, formed by the lowest points of the calcaneus, talonavicular joint, and head of the first metatarsal (normal values range from 120° to 130°) was also measured. These angles are greater in subjects who have flatfeet.

AOFAS average score improved from 72.2 points (range, 58–81) to 96.4 points (range, 87–100). Patient satisfaction was as follows: very high in 23 (41%); high in 28 (50%); low in 3 (5.4%); and very low in 2 (3.6%). When considering patient satisfaction, it is helpful to take into account that most patients had bilateral procedures.

Clinical correction of the deformity (**Fig. 6**) was evaluated using the Viladot footprint classification.[4] Most feet (94.8%) were classified as grade III or IV flatfoot before treatment, whereas 91.8% were normal or grade I or II flatfoot after surgery (**Fig. 7**). Preoperative and postoperative values are shown in **Table 1**.

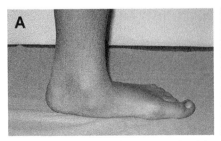
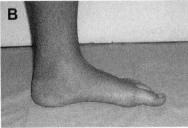

Fig. 6. Preoperative (A) and postoperative (B) aspect of a child's flatfoot treated by subtalar arthroereisis and Achilles tendon lengthening.

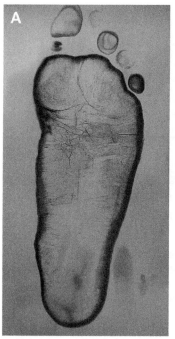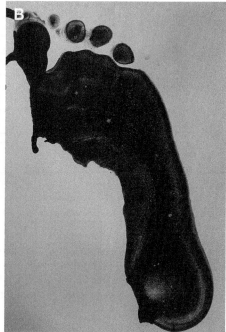

Fig. 7. (*A*) Preoperative footprint: grade III flatfoot. (*B*) Postoperative footprint: normal-grade I flatfoot.

Radiologic results were as follows: Mean Moreau-Costa-Bartani angle changed from 144.9° preoperative (136°–161°) to 127.5° postoperative (119°–135°) (**Fig. 8**). Mean Kite angle improved from 32.2° preoperative (26°–42°) to 19.3° postoperative (12°–28°). By the time the study was performed, the endorthesis had been removed in 37 feet—in 6 because of intolerance to the implant and in 31 it was removed without complications because the patients had reached the end of the growing period. The average angle loss in these feet after endorthesis removal was 0.8° in Moreau-Costa-Bartani angle and 0.3° in Kite angle (not statistically significant for both values) (**Fig. 9**).

Complications observed in this study included undercorrection in eight feet, over-correction in five, Achilles tendon contracture in four, pain at the sinus tarsi in four,

Table 1		
Preoperative and postoperative footprints according to Viladot		
	Preoperative	**Postoperative**
Grade 0	0 feet	31 feet
Grade I	0 feet	42 feet
Grade II	5 feet	16 feet
Grade III	39 feet	6 feet
Grade IV	53 feet	2 feet

From Viladot A. Surgical treatment of the child's flatfoot. Clin Orthop 1992;283:34–8; with permission.

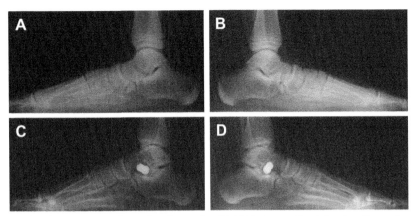

Fig. 8. (*A, B*) Preoperative lateral radiographs. (*C, D*) Postoperative lateral radiographs.

and peroneal tendon contracture in two. No cases of infection occurred. All cases with undercorrection had grade IV footprint before surgery and all improved clinically. The overcorrected cases were all asymptomatic. Four cases needed Achilles tendon lengthening (none had it lengthened when subtalar arthroereisis was performed). In

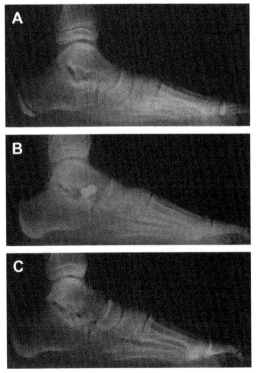

Fig. 9. (*A*) Preoperative lateral radiograph of an 8-year-old boy's flatfoot. (*B*) Postoperative lateral radiograph at 14 years of age. (*C*) Lateral radiograph at 17 years of age, 3 years after endorthesis removal. Note that there is no loss of correction.

all four feet with pain at sinus tarsi and the two with peroneal tendons contracture, symptoms disappeared after endorthesis removal.

DISCUSSION

Flexible flatfoot in children is a common condition that does not require surgery in most cases. However, some patients are symptomatic and, if they fulfill the inclusion criteria, require surgical treatment. Although numerous treatment options have been proposed, probably no single treatment is appropriate for every patient. Subtalar arthroereisis has proved to yield good mid- to long-term results.[3,4,11,13,15]

The purpose of arthroereisis is to relocate the talus properly over the calcaneus to allow remodeling of these bones and the subtalar joint during the remainder of the growing period.[9,24] This remodeling period should last at least 2 years. The foot reaches its bone maturity at age 14 to 15 years. Therefore, arthroereisis should best be performed before the age of 12, so that there are still two years for the remodeling period.

Achilles tendon lengthening is a surgical procedure that is very common in flatfoot treatment. Although some surgeons do not consider it necessary,[19] most publications about subtalar arthroereisis for flatfoot include Achilles tendon lengthening.[4,9,24,28,29] Gastrocnemius contracture is part of the pathologic anatomy of flatfoot and, in the authors' experience, is present in most cases. These investigators always decide preoperatively if Achilles lengthening is necessary. If ankle dorsiflexion is less than 10° while the knee is extended, they believe Achilles tendon lengthening is indicated.

Subtalar joint motion is usually diminished after arthroereisis, but the authors believe this should not be considered a complication. In fact, the purpose of arthroereisis is to limit the displacement of the talus over the calcaneus. Further investigation is required to evaluate if subtalar motion restriction recovers after implant removal. They also believe that supination of the foot in the early postoperative period is not a complication, because it resolves spontaneously 3 to 4 months after surgery.[24]

The authors advise endorthesis removal in all cases after the foot has achieved bone maturity (15–16 years of age). By that time, the implant has already performed its function and is no longer needed. Removal of the implant is a very simple procedure. In the authors' study, 38% of the feet had the endorthesis removed after completion of the foot's growth period. The average radiologic correction loss in these cases was minimal and not statistically significant.

In addition to the mentioned advantages of subtalar arthroereisis for flatfoot treatment (simple procedure, good results), this procedure has another important advantage: it allows further future surgery if needed. Osteotomies, arthrodesis, and soft tissue procedures are not hindered by subtalar arthroereisis.

SUMMARY

Subtalar arthroereisis, often combined with Achilles tendon lengthening, is a simple and effective way to treat flexible flatfoot in children. Mid- and long-term results are good, and the procedure does not prevent future treatments.

REFERENCES

1. Gould N, Schneider W, Ashikaga T. Epidemiological survey of foot problems in the continental United States: 1978–1979. Foot Ankle 1980;1:8–10.
2. García-Rodriguez A, Martin-Jimenez F, Carnero-Varo M, et al. Flexible flat feet in children: a real problem? Pediatrics 1999;103:84–95.

3. Smith SD, Millar EA. Arthroereisis by means of the subtalar polyethylene peg implant for correction of hindfoot pronation in children. Clin Orthop 1983;181:15–25.
4. Viladot A. Surgical treatment of the child's flatfoot. Clin Orthop 1992;283:34–8.
5. Chambers EF. An operation for the correction of flexible flat feet of adolescents. West J Surg Obstet Gynecol 1946;54:603–4.
6. Grice DS. An extra-articular arthrodesis of the subastragalar joint for correction of paralytic flat feet in children. J Bone Joint Surg Am 1952;34A(4):927–40.
7. Haraldsson S. Operative treatment of pes planovalgus staticus juvenilis. Acta Orthop Scand 1962;32:492–8.
8. Lelievre J. The valgus foot: current concepts and correction. Clin Orthop 1970;70: 43–55.
9. Zaret DI, Myerson MS. Arthroereisis of the subtalar joint. Foot Ankle Clin 2003;8: 605–17.
10. Needleman RL. Current topic review: subtalar arthroereisis for correction of flexible flatfoot. Foot Ankle Int 2005;26:336–46.
11. Subotnick S. The subtalar joint lateral extra-articular arthroereisis: a follow-up report. J Am Podiatry Assoc 1977;32:27–33.
12. Vedantam R, Capelli AM, Schoenecker PL. Subtalar arthroereisis for the correction of planovalgus foot in children with neuromuscular disorders. J Pediatr Orthop 1998;18:294–8.
13. Carranza-Bencano A, Zamora-Navas P, Fernández-Velazques JR. Viladot's operation in the treatment of the child's flatfoot. Foot Ankle Int 1997;18:544–9.
14. Black PR, Betts RP, Duckworth T, et al. The Viladot implant in flatfoot children. Foot Ankle Int 2000;21:478–81.
15. Giannini S. Operative treatment of the flatfoot: why and how. Foot Ankle Int 1998; 19:52–8.
16. Alvarez R. Calcaneo stop. Técnica personal original para el tratamiento quirúrgico del pie plano-valgo del niño y del adolescente jóven. In: Epeldegui T, editor. Pie plano y anomalías del antepié. Madrid, Spain: Madrid Vicente; 1995. p. 174–7.
17. Magnan B, Baldrighi C, Papadia D. Flatfeet: comparison of surgical techniques. Result of study group into retrograde endorthesis with calcaneus-stop. Ital J Pediatr Orthop 1997;13:28–33.
18. Nogarin L. Retrograde endorthesis. Ital J Pediatr Orthop 1997;13:34–9.
19. Roth S, Sestan B, Tudor A, et al. Minimally invasive calcaneo-stop method for idiopathic, flexible pes planovalgus in children. Foot Ankle Int 2007;28:991–5.
20. Vogler H. Subtalar joint blocking operations for pathological pronation syndromes. In: McGlamery ED, editor. Comprehensive textbook of foot surgery. Baltimore (MD): William & Wilkins; 1987. p. 466–82.
21. Mosca VS. Flexible flatfoot and tarsal coalition. In: Canale ST, editor. Orthopedic knowledge update: pediatrics 2. Chicago (IL): American Academy of Orthopaedic Surgeons; 2002. p. 215–7.
22. Kidner FC. The prehallux (accessory scaphoid) in relation to flat foot. J Bone Joint Surg Am 1929;11:831–7.
23. Molayem I, Persiani P, Marcovici LL, et al. Complications following correction of the planovalgus foot in cerebral palsy by arthroereisis. Acta Orthop Belg 2009; 75:374–9.
24. Gutiérrez PR, Herrera M. Giannini prosthesis for flatfoot. Foot Ankle Int 2005;26: 918–26.
25. Rocket AK, Mangum G, Mendicino SS. Bilateral intraosseous cystic formation in the talus: a complication of subtalar arthroereisis. J Foot Ankle Surg 1996;37: 421–5.

26. Siff TE, Granberry WM. Avascular necrosis of the talus following subtalar arthroer-
    eisis with a polyethylene endoprosthesis: a case report. Foot Ankle Int 2000;21:
    247–9.
27. Kuwada GT, Dockery GL. Complications following traumatic incidents with STA-
    peg procedures. J Foot Surg 1988;27:236–9.
28. Cicchinelli LD, Pascual-Huerta J, García-Carmona FJ, et al. Analysis of gastroc-
    nemius recession and medial column procedures as adjuncts in arthroereisis for
    the correction of pediatric pes planovalgus: a radiographic retrospective study.
    J Foot Ankle Surg 2008;47:385–91.
29. Nelson SC, Haycock DM, Little ER. Flexible flatfoot treatment with arthroereisis:
    radiographic improvement and child health survey analysis. J Foot Ankle Surg
    2004;43:144–55.

Adolescent Accessory Navicular

Zachary C. Leonard, MD[a,*], Paul T. Fortin, MD[a,b]

KEYWORDS

• Navicular • Accessory • Os • Foot

Accessory ossicles are common skeletal variations in the human foot and ankle. Historically, accessory ossicles are believed to be present in 18% to 30% of the population.[1,2] More recently, Coskun and colleagues[3] found accessory ossicles in 21.2% of patients. Accessory naviculars (ANs) are developmental in nature and originate from a secondary ossification center of the navicular bone. These ossicles may exist adjacent to the navicular or separated. Most accessory bones are asymptomatic radiographic findings, yet, a small portion can cause painful symptoms that necessitate treatment.[3,4]

The AN is the most common ossicle in the foot.[3] The first description is credited to Bauhin in 1605. Von Lushka, in 1858, furthered described its close association with the posterior tibial tendon and its jointlike attachment with the navicular bone proper. Over the years, many names have been coined for an AN, including accessory scaphoid, os tibiale, os tibiale externum, prehallux, os naviculare secundarium, and navicular secundum.[4–6] Geist[7] reported a 14% incidence in normal feet in 1914 and more recently Coskun and colleagues[3] found an 11.7% incidence in normal individuals. Grogan and colleagues[8] also stated up to a 13% incidence in the population. Other studies have reported between 2% and 14% incidence. McKusick[9] first reported inheritance of the ANs to be an autosomal dominant trait in 1994. Recently, an autosomal dominant pattern with incomplete penetrance has been demonstrated in studies by Kiter and colleagues[10] and Dobbs and Walton.[11]

A symptomatic AN must be differentiated from other pathologic causes of pain, notably occult fractures and degenerative arthritis.

ANATOMY AND EMBRYOLOGY

The navicular bone, also referred to as the scaphoid of the foot and os naviculare, is interposed in the foot between the head of the talus and the 3 cuneiforms. It has

[a] Department of Orthopaedics, William Beaumont Hospital, 3535 West Thirteen Mile Road, Medical Office Building Suite 744, Royal Oak, MI 48073, USA
[b] Orthopaedic Foot and Ankle Surgery, Oakland Orthopaedic Surgeons, 30575 Woodward Avenue, Royal Oak, Surgeons Suite 100, Royal Oak, MI 48073, USA
* Corresponding author.
E-mail address: zcleonard@gmail.com

Foot Ankle Clin N Am 15 (2010) 337–347
doi:10.1016/j.fcl.2010.02.004
1083-7515/10/$ – see front matter © 2010 Elsevier Inc. All rights reserved.

minimal articulation with the cuboid and is firmly bound through ligaments to the calcaneous. It takes a pyriform or pear shape with a long oblique axis directed inferior and medially. The round base is superolateral with an enlarged apex inferomedial. It has 4 surfaces; posterior, anterior, dorsal, and plantar with medial and lateral extremities. The navicular is flattened anteroposteriorly and is thicker dorsomedially. The medial end of the navicular is formed by a bony prominence, the navicular tuberosity, which is variable in size and provides the insertion for the posterior tibial tendon.[3]

The navicular is the last tarsal element to chondrify and its onset of ossification is variable and late in comparison to the other tarsal bones occurring at 2.7 to 4 years of age. The navicular bone normally has a single center of ossification.[3]

An AN is a congenital anomaly from which the tuberosity of the navicular develops from a secondary ossification center that fails to unite during childhood.[5] It is found on the medial aspect of the arch, posterior and medial to the tuberosity of the tarsal navicular bone. It is incorporated on the tuberosity of the navicular through insertional fibers of the posterior tibial tendon.[3] A typical AN is pyramidal in shape with its base anterior and apex posterior. Its connection to the tarsal navicular is usually fibrous or fibrocartilaginous and is described in detail in the following section. Its contour is variable as is its morphology. In 1925 Mouchet and Moutier described many of the roentgenographic morphologic variations.[3]

CLASSIFICATION

The original classification of ANs was proposed by Dwight in 1907.[12] He separated the sesamoid type (type 1). Since then, ANs have been further classified into 3 distinct types (**Fig. 1**).

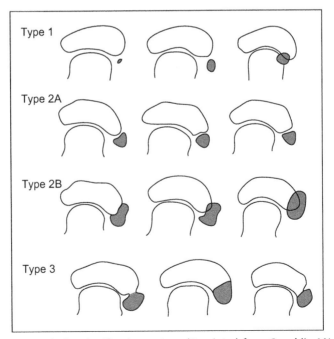

Fig. 1. Accessory navicular classification system. (*Reprinted from* Coughlin MJ. Sesamoids and accessory bones of the foot. In: Coughlin MJ, Mann RA, Saltzman CL, editors. Surgery of the foot and ankle. 8th edition. Philadelphia: Mosby; 2007. p. 592.)

Type 1 is a small (generally 2–3 mm in diameter) accessory bone within the posterior tibial tendon (PTT). It has no bony or cartilaginous attachment to the body of the tarsal navicular. It has been characterized as a sesamoid of the PTT. It is round or oval in shape and is located on the plantar aspect of the tendon near the calcaneonavicular ligament. It accounts for approximately 30% of ANs and is rarely symptomatic.

Type 2 AN has a fibrocartilaginous plate less than 2 mm in width with an irregular outline separating this tuberosity from the body of the navicular. This connection is referred to as a synchodrosis. This type is much larger in size (8–12 mm), and more triangular or heart-shaped in appearance. Type 2 are often symptomatic and can be mistaken as a fracture of the tuberosity. Type 2 is further differentiated into 2a and 2b based on the angle of attachment to the navicular. Type 2a connects with the talar process by a less acute angle resulting in a tension force that puts it at risk for avulsion injury. Type 2b attaches at an acute angle and sits more inferiorly leaving it susceptible to shearing forces.

Type 3 ANs are connected through a bony bridge, producing a cornuate (horny) navicular. Type 3 is theorized to represent an end stage of type 2. Type 3, like type 1 is rarely symptomatic. Type 2 and 3 ANs together comprise 70% of these deformities.[13]

An association has been made between AN and pes planus deformity. Flatfoot deformity is characterized by loss of the medial longitudinal arch, forefoot abduction, hindfoot eversion, and often Achilles tendon contracture.[14] Although much controversy persists, no causal relationship has been found. Prischasuk and Sinphurmsuk-skul[15] evaluated treatment of symptomatic AN and its relation to flat foot deformity. In their subset of patients, the calcaneal pitch angle in patients with symptomatic AN was significantly lower (14.8°) than in the normal subjects (21.4°). Thus, they were able to show an association between pes planus and symptomatic AN. However, according to Sullivan and Miller,[16] after review of patients with AN who had undergone simple excision compared with patients without AN, they found no difference in the medial longitudinal arch as measured by calcaneometatarsal angles. This led them to conclude that there is no evidence to support the opinion that an abnormal insertion of the PTT into an AN compromises the normal suspensory function of the PTT.

CLINICAL PRESENTATION

As is the case in many orthopedic pathologies, history and physical is paramount to the diagnosis of a painful AN. Medial foot pain can have a myriad of causes and it is necessary to evaluate each possibility thoroughly (**Box 1**). Most ANs become painful during childhood and early adulthood. Symptoms often begin in childhood from medial pressure of the accessory ossicle against the shoe. The most common complaints are pain and tenderness along the medial midfoot region. Swelling and erythema can also be present. These symptoms can be exacerbated by weight bearing, whether simply walking or running.[17] AN often becomes symptomatic in young athletes but also occurs in nonathletes following even a mild increase in athletic activity.[18] In addition, patients with symptomatic AN have difficulty tolerating narrow footwear.

IMAGING

Plain radiographs are the initial imaging modality and often the only imaging modality needed to diagnose an AN. Standard anteroposterior and lateral radiographs of the foot, along with a 45° external oblique view should be obtained when suspicious of an AN. Because the ossicle is often posterior and medial to the navicular proper,

Box 1
Differential diagnosis of medial midfoot pain

Accessory navicular

Fractured accessory navicular

Stress fracture: navicular

Stress fracture: metatarsals 1, 2

Stress fracture: medial/middle cuneiform

Posterior tibial tendonitis

Flexor hallucis longus tendonitis

Plantar fasciitis

Osteoarthritis, midfoot

Pes planovalgus

Kohler disease (navicular)

Tarsal tunnel syndrome

Peripheral vascular disease

the 45° external oblique is critical for visualization as it best assesses the medial tuberosity and the AN (**Fig. 2**). The standard internal oblique view can also be obtained to fully characterize the AN. Weight-bearing radiographs are recommended as they are more helpful in assessing associated capsuloligamentous instability and any

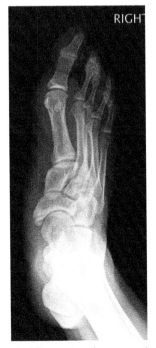

Fig. 2. Forty-five degree external oblique view demonstrating a type 2 AN.

concomitant pes planus. ANs should have rounded smooth borders as opposed to fractures, which have sharp ragged edges. Standard radiographs often allow identification and classification of the ossicle, but do not provide definitely a causal relationship to the patient with medial foot pain. Therefore, other imaging modalities along with a thorough physical examination are sometimes necessary.[19]

Technetium bone scans can be used to assess ANs. Often bone scans are ordered when a fracture is suspected. Increased uptake is seen with avulsion tuberosity fractures and ANs. Sella and colleagues[13] evaluated 9 patients with symptomatic type 2 ANs. These patients showed focal uptake in the AN on technetium scans. Furthermore, the bone scans were specific to the symptomatic side in patients with bilateral AN.

Magnetic resonance can help to differentiate an AN from a tuberosity fracture by revealing the presence or absence of bone edema.[19] Miller and colleagues[20] evaluated 14 feet (7 patients) with radiographically documented type 2 ANs and unilateral foot pain. Of those patients, 5 had focal pain in the region of the AN. All 5 had an abnormal bone marrow edema pattern of the AN on magnetic resonance imaging.

Computed tomography can be helpful to delineate the bony anatomy more clearly; this test is often ordered when fracture is suspected and plain films have poor visualization or are inconclusive (**Fig. 3**). Ultrasound is not often used for diagnosis of an AN. However, it can be useful in distinguishing between complete or partial separation through the synchondrosis and rupture of attenuation of the posterior tibial tendon in patients with suspected injury to the AN or PTT.[21]

CONSERVATIVE MANAGEMENT

As with many orthopedic conditions, initial efforts should be nonoperative for a symptomatic AN. This includes relieving pressure on the medial midfoot and decreasing inflammation. In many cases, identification of the ossicle and reassurance may be all the treatment that is needed. Shoe-wear modification should be first-line treatment. Wider, more comfortable shoes that off-load the medial midfoot can be obtained over the counter or prescription orthoses can be customized for the patient. Activity modification, such as limiting or stopping any strenuous activities that cause the AN to become symptomatic can be used for initial treatment. Casting can be used to prevent repetitive microtrauma either directly or from pull of the posterior tibial tendon. Nonsteroidal antiinflammatorie drugs can be used as an adjunctive treatment of pain relief and to decrease swelling associated with an inflamed AN. Corticosteroid

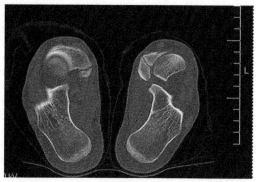

Fig. 3. Computed tomography images of foot demonstrating bilateral type 2 AN.

injections can be used as a treatment modality. However, this modality should be used with caution as it may weaken the posterior tibial tendon and lead to subsequent rupture.[22]

SURGICAL TREATMENT

When conservative measures fail, surgery is indicated. There are multiple surgical treatment options described in the literature. They vary from simple excision, to excision and rerouting of the posterior tibial tendon under the navicular, excision and restoring the continuity of the PTT, percutaneous drilling, or arthrodesis of the accessory ossicle.

Kidner[23,24] emphasized that an abnormal insertion of the tendon into the ossicle changes the leverage of the tendon, interfering with normal tarsal mechanics and producing a weakness of the longitudinal arch and a resultant painful flat foot. To remedy this problem, Kidner proposed a procedure that consists of excising the AN and rerouting the tibialis posterior tendon into a more plantar position to restore the normal line of pull in 1929 and 1933. Leonard and colleagues[25] supported the use of this operation. They believed, as Kidner did, that PTT insertion into the accessory ossicle deprives the foot of a portion of its medial sling, and flat foot may result. Leonard and colleagues' paper in 1965 outlined their surgical technique and reported "most satisfactorily, producing a good arch, correcting the heel valgus, and controlling the progression of the hallux valgus." Ray and Goldberg[26] used this procedure in 29 patients with an AN or navicular beaks. Only 3 poor results were reported, all in the navicular beak group (type 3 AN) and no poor results in the AN group (type 2). Veitch[27] reviewed a series of 21 patients who had undergone a Kidner procedure for symptomatic type 2 and type 3 AN. Although no patient rated their result as poor, no radiographic or photographic improvement of the arch could be documented in any patient and all but 2 patients noted no change in their arch. He concluded that the Kidner operation is a successful method of treatment, but that the success is related to removal of the bony prominence on the medial aspect of the foot and its mechanical irritation than to the correction of the pronated foot as a result of the PTT transfer.

Simple excision of the AN is well published in the literature. This procedure was first suggested by Geist in 1925.[7] Sella and colleagues,[13] as mentioned earlier, had a series of 9 patients with type 2 AN treated surgically with excision with repair of the PTT, but no attempt to transfer the tendon insertion plantarly with good results in all. In 1984, Macnicol and Voutsinas[28] reported on the results of 26 patients treated by Kidner procedures and 21 patients treated with mere excision. Patients with more severe pes planus were preferentially treated with Kidner operations. Symptoms were relieved equally in both groups. However, radiographic improvement in arch height occurred in operative and nonoperative feet particularly in young patients. This confirms that the growing foot typically develops a higher arch as it matures.[29]

In addition, Grogan and colleagues[8] reported on a series of 25 feet with symptomatic AN that were refractory to conservative management. All patients underwent excision by splitting the tendon longitudinally and elevating dorsally and plantarly to provide exposure of the AN without any attempt to reroute the posterior tibial tendon. All were completely relieved of preoperative pain. Kopp and Marcus[30] reviewed 14 consecutive patients with type 2 AN that failed conservative management. Excision was performed by exposing the dorsal aspect of the PTT and elevating it off the AN. A periosteal elevator was used to aid in delineating the AN attachment to the main navicular bone. The plantar aspect of the PTT was left undisturbed as the AN was shelled out. The dorsal tendinous insertion of the PTT was sutured to the periosteum of connective tissue flap with multiple sutures. At final follow-up, 13 of 14 feet were without any pain and all had no activity restrictions. More recently, Jasiewicz and colleagues[31] reviewed 22 patients with a mean age of 14.1 years who underwent simple excision of the symptomatic AN. At a mean follow-up of 5.6 years, only 1 patient had persistent pain and no relief. All patients were able to single heel-rise pre- and postoperatively. The investigators concluded that simple excision effectively reduces pain and restores physical function. Micheli and colleagues[32] recently published a modification to simple excision using parallel incisions at the superior and inferior borders of the PTT and leaving the proximal and distal longitudinal fibers attached. The central third of the PTT complex is elevated and the AN is rongeured out. The PTT complex and its associated periosteum are then sutured inferior to the body of the navicular, and the inferior leaf of the periosteal flap is reapproximated superiorly. The tendon fibers inserting on the navicular are not disturbed. Thirteen feet with an average age of 13.5 years were treated with this procedure. Eleven reported excellent results and 2 reported good results. The advantage of this technique is that the PTT remains intact, decreasing the period of immobilization compared with the Kidner procedure.

Senses and colleagues[33] treated symptomatic type 2 AN by excision and restoring the continuity of the PTT. They noted that the PTT ended at the AN and another tendon, PTT secondarius, originating from the navicular bone. After excision of the AN and the slip, the PTT secondarius was detached from the navicular and sutured to the main portion of the PTT. All patients (8/8) healed uneventfully and were able to perform the single heel-rise test. Although clinical preoperative evaluation revealed flattening of the medial longitudinal arch, no improvement in the medial arch was seen postoperatively. Thus, they were not able to demonstrate any clear association between ANs and flat feet.

A technique of percutaneous drilling of symptomatic type 2 ANs in a series of young athletes to induce or accelerate bone union has shown favorable results by Nakayama and colleagues[34] Thirty of 31 (96.8%) reported excellent (79.4%) or good (19.4%) results in this series even though bone union could only be confirmed on 58% of the 31 feet. In this technique, a 1.0-mm Kirschner wire is introduced percutaneously from the posterior aspect of the AN prominence to the primary navicular through the synchondrosis at 5 to 7 different points. The investigators noted that this method is minimally invasive, easy, economical, and without complications, and should therefore be used before open procedures. Further studies are needed to validate this method.

Another relatively new treatment method is arthrodesis of the accessory ossicle with the navicular proper. Malicky and colleagues[35] used a modification of the Kidner procedure using fusion. They removed the medial midfoot prominence, fused the primary and AN bones, and advanced the PTT distally and plantarly. The soft tissue interval (synchondrosis) is excised, then the bones are arthrodesed using one or two 2.7- or 3.5-mm lag screws. In this method, the native PTT attachment to bone is left intact and healing occurs across a reliable bony surfaces. Scott and colleagues[36] prospectively evaluated fusion versus excision with advancement of the PTT of 20 patients with symptomatic type 2 AN. Decisions for treatment were made intraoperatively based on the size of the ossicle. If the ossicle was large enough to accommodate screws, then a fusion was undertaken. On the contrary, if the ossicle was small, then it was excised and the PTT advanced. The arthrodesis group had a trend toward improved (American Orthopaedic Foot and Ankle Society (AOFAS) scores compared with excision. It should be noted that adjunctive, joint-sparing corrective procedures in all patients with associated pes planus was performed, irrespective of the surgical management of the symptomatic type 2 AN. In another recent study by Chung and Chu[37] in 2009, 34 feet were analyzed radiographically and clinically after fusion of painful type 2 AN. Six patients developed nonunions and defined outcomes as poor. The other 28 (82%) patients obtained bony union and were able to participate in sporting activities. They concluded that although there were a few nonunions, fusion overall showed a low rate of complications and a high rate of patient satisfaction.

AUTHORS' PREFERRED TREATMENT

When a symptomatic AN is unresponsive to nonoperative modalities, surgical intervention is indicated. Assessment of foot alignment, flexibility, and the patient's primary source of discomfort are important factors. Not uncommonly, these patients can have isolated medial midfoot pain that is caused by increased medial arch strain after concomitant planovalgus deformity and/or gastrocsoleus tightness and the AN is incidental. The size of the AN, shape and size of the native navicular bone, and concomitant foot malalignment are the primary factors in the surgical decision-making process.

In patients with a small symptomatic AN, a native navicular that is normal in shape, and no significant planovalgus deformity, simple excision is reasonable. In most circumstances, this can be accomplished without significantly disrupting the continuity of the posterior tibial tendon. A patient may infrequently have a small symptomatic AN with a large cornuate-shaped native navicular with significant prominence on the medial midfoot. In this circumstance, partial excision of the prominence of the cornuate-shaped native navicular and excision of the AN with advancement of the posterior tibial tendon is indicated.

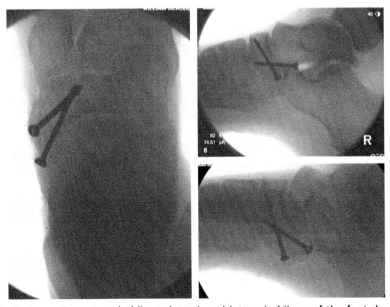

Fig. 4. Postoperative external oblique, lateral, and internal oblique of the foot shown in **Fig. 2** after undergoing excision of the synchondrosis and fusion with 2.7 cortical screw fixation.

In patients with concomitant planovalgus deformity and/or gastrocsoleus tightness, the treatment should in general be primarily directed toward diminishing medial arch strain. Often this by itself sufficiently relieves the discomfort associated with the AN. The specific treatment regimen has to be individualized based on radiographic and clinical parameters of deformity and flexibility of the foot. The specifics of flatfoot correction are not the intent of this article nor can they be generalized to every patient with a symptomatic AN and concomitant planovalgus.

Patients with a large AN with significant prominence on the medial midfoot often have an associated cornuate-shaped native navicular bone. If no significant planovalgus deformity exists, the authors prefer the technique described by Malicky and colleagues[35] that involves segmental excision/osteotomy of the synchondrosis to diminish the overall width of the navicular and fusion of the AN to the native navicular with two 2.7-mm lag screws to provide for rotational control (**Fig. 4**). If concomitant planovalgus exists, this is corrected simultaneously if it is felt there will be persistent increased medial arch strain with fusion alone.

SUMMARY

Accessory tarsal navicular is a common anomaly in the human foot. It should be in the differential of medial foot pain. A proper history and physical, along with imaging modalities, can lead to the diagnosis. Often, classification of the ossicle and amount of morbidity guide treatment. Nonsurgical measures can provide relief. A variety of surgical procedures have been used with good results. Our preferred method is excision for small ossicles and segmental fusion after removal of the synchondrosis for large ossicles. In addition, pes planovalgus deformities need to be addressed concomitantly.

REFERENCES

1. Shands AR, Wentz IJ. Congenital anomalies, accessory bones, and osteochondritis in the foot of 850 children. Surg Clin North Am 1953;33:1643–66.
2. Kruse RW, Chen J. Accessory bones of the foot: clinical significance. Mil Med 1995;160:464–7.
3. Coskun N, Yuksel M, Cevener M, et al. Incidence of accessory ossicles and sesamoid bones in the feet: a radiographical study of the Turkish subjects. Surg Radiol Anat 2009;31(1):19–24.
4. Ugolini P, Raikin S. The accessory navicular. Foot Ankle Clin 2004;9(1):165–80.
5. Coughlin MJ. Sesamoids and accessory bones of the foot. In: Coughlin MJ, Mann RA, Saltzman CL, editors. Surgery of the foot and ankle. 8th edition. Philadelphia: Mosby; 2007. p. 531–610.
6. Sarrafian SK. Anatomy of the foot and ankle. Philadelphia: JB Lippincott; 1983.
7. Geist ES. The accessory scaphoid bone. J Bone Joint Surg 1925;7:570–4.
8. Grogan D, Gasser S, Ogden J. The painful accessory navicular: a clinical and histopathological study. Foot Ankle 1989;10:164–9.
9. McKusick VA. Mendelian inheritance in man. Baltimore (MD): The John Hopkins University Press; 1994.
10. Kiter E, Erduran M, Gunal I. Inheritance of the accessory navicular bone. Arch Orthop Trauma Surg 2000;120:582–3.
11. Dobbs MB, Walton T. Autosomal dominant transmission of accessory navicular. Iowa Orthop J 2004;24:84–5.

12. Dwight T. Variations of the bones of the hands and feet: a clinical atlas. Philadelphia: JB Lippincott; 1907.
13. Sella EJ, Lawson JP, Ogden JA. The accessory navicular synchondrosis. Clin Orthop 1986;209:280–5.
14. Blackman AJ, Blevins JJ, Sangeorzan BJ, et al. Cadaveric flatfoot model: ligament attenuation and Achilles tendon overpull. J Orthop Res 2009;27(12):1547–54.
15. Prichasuk S, Sinphurmsukskul O. Kidner procedure for symptomatic accessory navicular and its relation to pes planus. Foot Ankle Int 1995;16:500–3.
16. Sullivan JA, Miller WA. The relationship of the accessory navicular to the development of the flat foot. Clin Orthop 1979;144:233–7.
17. Mygind H. The accessory tarsal scaphoid; clinical features and treatment. Acta Orthop Scand 1953;23(2):142–51.
18. Sella EJ, Lawson JP. Biomechanics of the accessory navicular synchondrosis. Foot Ankle 1987;8:156–63.
19. Johnson TR, Steinbach LS. Accessory navicular. In: Johnson TR, Steinbach LS, editors. Essentials of musculoskeletal imaging. Rosemont (IL): AAOS; 2004. p. 574–6.
20. Miller TT, Staron RB, Feldman F, et al. The symptomatic accessory tarsal navicular bone: assessment with MRI imaging. Radiology 1995;195:849–53.
21. Yeung-Jen C, Wen-Wei R, Liang S. Degeneration of the accessory navicular synchondrosis presenting as rupture of the posterior tibial tendon. J Bone Joint Surg Am 1997;79(12):1791–8.
22. Strayhorn G, Puhl J. The symptomatic accessory navicular bone. J Fam Pract 1982;15(1):59–64.
23. Kidner FC. The pre-hallux (accessory scaphoid) in its relation to the flat-foot. J Bone Joint Surg 1929;11:831–7.
24. Kidner FC. The prehallux in relation to flat-foot. J Am Med Assoc 1933;101(20):1539–42.
25. Leonard MH, Gonzales S, Breck LW, et al. Lateral transfer of the posterior tibial tendon in certain selected cases of pes plano valgus (Kidner operation). Clin Orthop 1965;40:139–44.
26. Ray S, Goldberg VM. Surgical treatment of the accessory navicular. Clin Orthop 1983;177:61–6.
27. Veitch JM. Evaluation of the Kidner procedure in treatment of symptomatic accessory tarsal scaphoid. Clin Orthop 1978;131:210–3.
28. Macnicol MF, Voutsinas S. Surgical treatment of the symptomatic accessory navicular. J Bone Joint Surg Br 1984;66:218–26.
29. Jones BS. Flatfoot: a preliminary report of an operation for severe cases. J Bone Joint Surg Br 1975;57:279–82.
30. Kopp FJ, Marcus RE. Clinical outcome of surgical treatment of the symptomatic accessory navicular. Foot Ankle Int 2004;25:27–30.
31. Jasiewicz B, Potaczek T, Kacki W, et al. Results of simple excision technique in the surgical treatment of symptomatic accessory navicular bones. Foot Ankle Surg 2008;14:57–61.
32. Micheli LJ, Nielson JH, Ascani C, et al. Treatment of painful accessory navicular: a modification to simple excision. Foot Ankle Spec 2008;1:214–7.
33. Senses I, Kiter E, Gunal I. Restoring the continuity of the tibialis posterior tendon in the treatment of symptomatic accessory navicular with flat feet. J Orthop Sci 2004;9:408–9.
34. Nakayama S, Sugimoto K, Takakura Y, et al. Percutaneous drilling of symptomatic accessory navicular in young athletes. Am J Sports Med 2005;33:531–5.

35. Malicky ES, Levine DS, Sangeorzan BJ. Modification of the Kidner procedure with fusion of the primary and accessory navicular bones. Foot Ankle Int 1999;20: 53–4.
36. Scott AT, Sabesan VJ, Saluta JR, et al. Fusion versus excision of the symptomatic type II accessory navicular: a prospective study. Foot Ankle Int 2009;30:10–5.
37. Chung JW, Chu IT. Outcome of fusion of a painful accessory navicular to the primary navicular. Foot Ankle Int 2009;30(2):106–9.

Tarsal Coalitions

Htwe Zaw, FRCS (Tr&Orth)[a],*,
James D.F. Calder, MD, FRCS (Tr&Orth), FFSEM(UK)[b]

KEYWORDS

• Tarsal coalition • Cause • Diagnosis • Management

A tarsal coalition is an aberrant union between 2 or more tarsal bones and can be classified as osseous (synostosis) or nonosseous (cartilaginous [synchondrosis] or fibrous [syndesmosis]). This union may be complete or partial and the joints in the hindfoot and midfoot are most commonly affected. The resulting abnormal articulation presents as a noncorrectable flat foot, usually during adolescence, leading to accelerated degeneration within adjacent joints. An understanding of the condition and presenting symptoms enable the clinician to correctly diagnose and initiate appropriate treatment. This review discusses the evidence-based literature on the cause, diagnosis, and current management of tarsal coalition.

HISTORICAL REVIEW

Tarsal coalition is a phenomenon that has been known for many years. Archeological specimens dating from 900 to 1000 AD have confirmed their presence in the ruins of a Mayan temple in Guatemala[1] and a pre-Columbian Indian skeleton in Ohio.[2] More recently in 2005, Silva[3] presented 2 cases of nonosseous calcaneonavicular coalition in older specimens recovered from Portuguese burial sites dating from between the late Neolithic and early Bronze Age, circa 3600 to 2000 BC.

The first description of a tarsal coalition is attributed to Buffon[4] in 1769. This French naturalist attempted the monumental task of encapsulating the sum of human knowledge about the natural world in a single book, *Histoire naturelle, générale et particulière*. However, Cruveilhier[5] is credited with performing the first anatomic description of a calcaneonavicular coalition in 1829. This was later followed by descriptions of talocalcaneal and talonavicular coalitions by Zuckerlandl[6] and Anderson.[7] In 1880, Holl[8] tentatively suggested a relationship between tarsal coalition and peroneal spasm. This association was later supported by work from Slomann,[9] Badgley,[10] and Harris and Beath.[11]

The first radiologic depiction of a tarsal coalition took place in 1898 by Kirmisson,[12] only 3 years after Roentgen discovered x-rays. In 1921, Slomann[9] demonstrated the

[a] Department of Trauma and Orthopaedic Surgery, Basingstoke and North Hampshire Hospitals NHS Foundation Trust, Aldermaston Road, Basingstoke RG24 9NA, UK
[b] Imperial College School of Medicine Science and Technology, Charing Cross Hospital, London W6 8RF, UK
* Corresponding author.
E-mail address: htwe@hotmail.com

Foot Ankle Clin N Am 15 (2010) 349–364
doi:10.1016/j.fcl.2010.02.003
foot.theclinics.com

usefulness of a 45° lateral oblique radiograph in identifying calcaneonavicular coalitions. This enabled him to explain the association between hindfoot rigidity, marked flat foot, and tarsal coalition. Badgley[10] demonstrated this in 1927 by successfully resecting 2 osseous calcaneonavicular coalitions. In 1934, Korvin[13] first described the 45° axial or ski-jump view of the heel to visualize talocalcaneal coalitions. This technique was later popularized by Harris and Beath[11] in their classic paper from 1948, in which they published a series of peroneal spastic flatfoot in association with talocalcaneal coalition. The term peroneal spastic flatfoot is no longer used, as it describes only one of several clinical presentations of tarsal coalition and the condition may exist in the absence of a coalition.[14,15]

Other tarsal coalitions have been described but are less common. Calcaneocuboid coalition was first recognized by Holland[16] in 1918. Waugh[17] and Lusby[18] first reported cubonavicular and naviculocuneiform coalitions, respectively. Multiple coalitions involving several tarsal bones have also been reported.[19,20]

INCIDENCE

The documented overall incidence of tarsal coalition is 1% or less.[21–23] However, it is commonly agreed that the true incidence is much higher as coalitions go undiagnosed in the asymptomatic and nonosseous subtypes.[24–26] Solomon and colleagues[27] studied 100 cadaveric feet using computed tomography (CT) scanning and subsequent dissection, and concluded that the incidence of talocalcaneal coalition was as high as 12.7%. The joints most commonly affected are talocalcaneal and calcaneonavicular, which account for approximately 90% of cases. Stormont and Peterson[21] performed a review of 314 cases of tarsal coalition from 11 studies, revealing the proportion of talocalcaneal coalition to be 48.1%, calcaneonavicular was 43.6%, both talonavicular and calcaneocuboid were 1.3% each, and an unspecified group made up the remaining 5.7%. Of the 2 most common types, calcaneonavicular coalitions tend to be overwhelmingly nonosseous, whereas talonavicular coalitions have a more even distribution of the 3 histologic subtypes.[25]

The incidence of bilateral tarsal coalition varies in the literature but is generally believed to be 50% or more.[28–30] Stormont and Peterson[21] found 68% of calcaneonavicular coalitions were bilateral. Leonard[31] reported a bilateral rate of 80% in 31 cases of tarsal coalition, most of which were also calcaneonavicular. He also found equal sex distribution but subsequent studies indicate a slight male preponderance.[21,30] Although no racial or geographic variation in incidence of calcaneonavicular or talocalcaneal coalitions have been demonstrated, a relatively large number of naviculocuneiform coalitions have been reported from Japan.[32–34] Furthermore, Burnett and Case[35] analyzed skeletal remains from African and European ancestry. They found naviculocuneiform coalitions were statistically more prevalent in the South African Bantu population than in European ancestry. This suggests the possibility of population variation with certain types of tarsal coalition.

ETIOLOGY

Tarsal coalitions can be congenital or acquired. Acquired coalitions may result from trauma, surgery, arthritis, infection and neoplasia.[15,36] They are rare and more prevalent in the adult population. Congenital tarsal coalitions are far more common and usually seen in the adolescent group. They originate from the failure of differentiation and segmentation of embryonic mesenchyme, inherited in an autosomal dominant pattern.[31,37–40]

In 1896, Pfitzner[41] proposed that tarsal coalitions were caused by the incorporation of accessory ossicles into the major adjacent tarsal bones. His primary evidence was that the accessory ossicles appear at the sites where many tarsal coalitions occur, such as the os sustentaculum proprium in the middle facet and the os calcaneus secundarius in the calcaneonavicular space. This idea received support from the work of Slomann,[9] Badgely,[10] and Chambers and colleagues.[42]

Harris[37] demonstrated the presence of a talocalcaneal coalition in the fetus in 1955 and confirmed their embryologic origin. This effectively eliminated Pfitzner's theory, as accessory ossicles could not have yet developed in the fetus. Earlier in 1890, Leboucq[38] suggested that tarsal coalitions resulted from the failure of differentiation and segmentation of primitive embryonic mesenchyme. The findings by Harris corroborated this and subsequent work by other investigators also support a mesenchymal defect as the cause.[22,28,39] Furthermore, there is strong evidence in the literature to suggest that an inherited defect in genetic coding is responsible for the development of tarsal coalition.[29–31,40] The inheritance pattern is believed to be autosomal dominant with high penetrance. Wray and Herndon[40] demonstrated a calcaneonavicular coalition in 3 successive generations of males with unaffected mother and sister. Based on Mendelian patterns of inheritance, they concluded that a specific gene mutation, behaving in an autosomal dominant manner, was responsible for calcaneonavicular coalitions. Leonard[31] reviewed 98 first-degree relatives of 31 index patients with confirmed tarsal coalitions. He found 33% of the parents and 46% of the siblings had radiographic evidence of tarsal coalition, all of which were asymptomatic. He concluded that tarsal coalition was a unifactorial disorder of autosomal dominant inheritance. He also suggested the condition had near full penetrance as he demonstrated a high rate of bilateral coalitions in parents (83%) and siblings (85%), similar to that found in the index group (80%).

Plotkin[43] presented a case of calcaneonavicular coalition in monozygotic twins and suggested that the inheritance of tarsal coalition is more complicated than a simple Mendelian pattern. He proposed that it is likely to be a defect in a general joint development gene as part of a complex polygenic system responsible for overall limb development. This would account for the findings in Leonard's study, which showed different sites of coalition in the relatives than those found in the index group. Syndromes that may present with tarsal coalition include carpal coalition, symphalangism, arthrogryposis, fibula hemimelia, Apert syndrome, and Nievergelt-Pearlman syndrome.[15,30,31,36] The relative contribution of an environmental congenital defect, an error in mesenchymal differentiation, or an inherited genetic defect that leads to the formation of tarsal coalition is still uncertain. The fact that a genetic component exists should alert the clinician to asymptomatic siblings and close relatives with the condition.

PATHOPHYSIOLOGY

The normal subtalar joint undergoes rotational and gliding movements during stance and walking. The axis of the joint is 42° from the horizontal plane and 16° medial to a line extending from the center of the calcaneus to the midpoint between the first and second metatarsals.[44] During the stance phase, the subtalar joint rotates from 4° of external to 6° of internal rotation, which accommodates the external rotation of the tibia.[45] The lack of internal rotation in the subtalar joint from a coalition causes the calcaneocuboid and talonavicular joints to compensate. This causes a planovalgus deformity with flattening of the longitudinal arch and forefoot abduction. Adaptive shortening and spasm of the peroneal tendons produces the so-called peroneal spastic flatfoot. Prolonged restriction of subtalar motion eventually leads to arthrosis of the posterior facet, as well as the midtarsal and ankle joints.

During foot dorsiflexion, the gliding motion of the subtalar joint is recruited.[46] The calcaneus glides forward on the talus until it is restricted by capsular ligaments. At the end of dorsiflexion the talonavicular and calcaneocuboid joints glide superiorly. A reduction in subtalar glide as a result of the presence of a coalition leads to compensatory hingelike movement at the talonavicular joint. The navicular overrides the talar head at maximum dorsiflexion, repeatedly elevating the dorsal capsule and creating a traction spur.[15,47] This is believed to be the mechanism behind talar beaking seen on lateral radiographs (**Fig. 1**).

PRESENTATION

Patients with tarsal coalition usually present with symptoms during the second decade of life. Those younger than 8 years may present with foot fatigue while the coalition remains fibrocartilaginous. Symptoms are more likely to manifest as the coalition progressively ossifies, altering the kinematics of the joint.[15,23,48] The onset of symptoms can be variable as different types of coalition ossify at different stages. The relatively uncommon talonavicular coalition ossifies earliest around 3 to 5 years of age, calcaneonavicular coalitions ossify between 8 and 12 years, and talocalcaneal coalitions usually between 12 and 16 years.[49,50]

Pain is the most common presenting symptom, followed by valgus deformity and subtalar stiffness. The primary source of pain may be attributed to ligament strain, peroneal spasm, sinus tarsi syndrome, or subtalar arthrosis. Microfractures and histologic signs of normal bone remodeling have been identified at the coalition-bone interface and are likely to be the pain generators via periosteal nerve fibers.[51] The absence of nerve tissue in histologic analysis of resected nonosseus coalitions argues against the abnormal coalition tissue acting as the primary pain generator.[51] Pain can be localized to the sinus tarsi in a calcaneonavicular coalition or the medial subtalar joint in a talocalcaneal coalition. However, it is often diffuse and insidious, exacerbated by strenuous activity or following an ankle sprain that is slow to resolve. An episode of trauma may act as the trigger to a previously dormant coalition and may be the case in patients presenting in adulthood. A history of recurrent sprains should alert the clinician to the possible diagnosis of tarsal coalition. Variability in the level of pain, stiffness, and deformity on presentation reflects the degree of restriction in

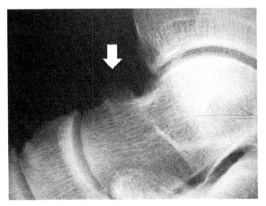

Fig. 1. Talar beaking on lateral radiograph.

subtalar motion from different types of coalition. Talocalcaneal coalitions within the middle facet create the greatest loss of subtalar motion and the most obvious valgus deformity.[15,30,52]

Physical examination can reveal a rigid valgus hindfoot with forefoot abduction, although a neutral or varus hindfoot does not exclude the diagnosis.[53] Loss of subtalar motion may be determined by a reverse Coleman block test: the patient's foot is supinated by raising the medial border of the forefoot using a block and keeping the heel and lateral border in contact with the floor. If the heel valgus remains uncorrected, the hindfoot is no longer mobile. In addition, a decrease in the normal external rotation of the tibia is observed, reflected by absent outward rotation of the patella. A simpler way to assess restricted subtalar motion is to ask the patient to walk on the outer borders of their feet, which may be difficult or uncomfortable to perform. A single-heel raise test will reveal the absence of normal heel varus. Tenderness may be elicited over the sinus tarsi or the middle facet, just distal to the medial malleolus. A reduction in passive eversion and inversion are commonly seen in all types of tarsal coalition. Although it is vital to compare the findings with the contralateral foot, there should be a high index of suspicion for the presence of bilateral coalitions. Associated peroneal muscle spasm on forced inversion is suggestive but not diagnostic of a coalition.[14,15]

IMAGING
Conventional Radiography

Initial evaluation of a patient with possible tarsal coalition begins with the acquisition of 3 images: anteroposterior, lateral, and 45° oblique weight-bearing views of the feet. It is well recognized that tarsal coalitions can be difficult to diagnose using conventional radiography, especially talocalcaneal coalitions,[30,36] because of bone overlap, obliquity of the coalition, and coalitions of fibrocartilaginous origin.[15] Instead, assessment is limited to the recognition of secondary signs suggestive of an occult coalition. An elongated anterior calcaneal process on the lateral view, known as the anteater nose sign, may suggest the presence of a calcaneonavicular coalition (**Fig. 2**). This radiographic sign may not be apparent in young children before the age of 8 years as the coalition has yet to ossify. The 45° oblique view of the foot demonstrates a calcaneonavicular coalition in 90% to 100% of cases (**Fig. 3**).[9,22,28,50] Of these, only 10% demonstrate a frank osseous bridge; the remainder demonstrate secondary signs. These include a decrease in the calcaneonavicular gap, irregular sclerotic cortices, an elongated lateral navicular as it approaches the anterior calcaneus (reverse

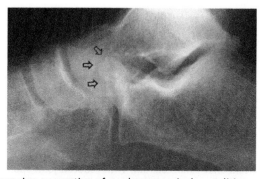

Fig. 2. Anteater nose sign suggestive of a calcaneonavicular coalition.

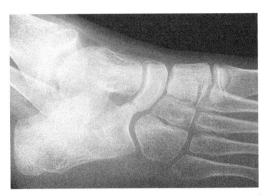

Fig. 3. Calcaneonavicular coalition visualized on 45° oblique radiograph.

anteater sign), and hypoplasia of the lateral talar head (**Fig. 4**).[36,54,55] Lysack and Fenton[26] used these secondary signs on plain radiographs to demonstrate a high prevalence of nonosseous calcaneonavicular coalitions (5.6%) in 460 patients presenting to the emergency department with acute foot pain. They suggested that many of the coalitions found did not require further evaluation with CT or magnetic resonance imaging (MRI) because most were asymptomatic.

Talocalcaneal coalitions are best seen with an additional axial or ski-jump view popularized by Harris and Beath.[11] This is taken with the patient standing on the cassette and dorsiflexing 10° at the ankle. Harris and Beath originally recommended a 45° beam from behind the heel. They later expanded the views to include beam angles of 30°, 35°, and 45° to visualize the subtalar joint clearly. An osseous coalition in the middle facet obliterates that part of the joint, whereas a nonosseous coalition produces irregular cortices and a dysplastic sustentaculum tali.

Lateur[56] described the C sign seen in talocalcaneal coalitions on the lateral radiograph, a circular density composed of the talar dome and inferior margin of the sustentaculum tali (**Fig. 5**). In 2000, Sakellariou and colleagues[57] concluded a 98% sensitivity and specificity using the C sign to diagnose talocalcaneal coalitions. They compared lateral radiographs of 20 patients with suspected talocalcaneal coalitions on clinical assessment and conventional radiography with 22 asymptomatic volunteers. The diagnosis was confirmed on subsequent CT scanning. However, a retrospective review by Brown and colleagues[58] of 48 patients with lateral foot radiographs and CT scans for atraumatic indications, found the C sign to be neither sensitive nor specific for talocalcaneal coalition, and only specific for a flatfoot deformity.

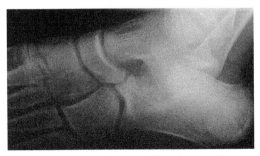

Fig. 4. Nonosseus calcaneonavicular coalition with reduced joint space, sclerotic cortices, elongated lateral navicular (reverse anteater sign) and hypoplasia of the lateral talar head.

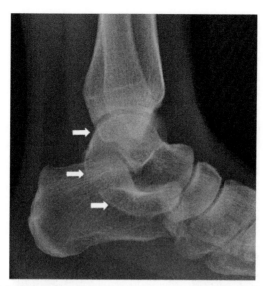

Fig. 5. C sign on lateral radiograph suggestive of a talocalcaneal coalition.

Talar beaking is seen most commonly in talocalcaneal coalition but also occurs in calcaneonavicular coalition (see **Fig. 1**). It is believed to be the result of repeated elevation and traction of the dorsal capsule of the talonavicular joint, as the navicular overrides the talar head during foot dorsiflexion.[15,47] Other secondary signs suggestive of a talocalcaneal coalition include a short talar neck with a concave inferior surface, narrow posterior facet of the subtalar joint and failure to see the middle facet.[36,54] Conventional radiography in the initial consultation is also useful in identifying other causes of peroneal spasm, such as an inflammatory arthropathy, a subtle cavus deformity, or infection of the tarsus leading to ankylosis.[15] Despite the secondary signs on conventional radiographs, most patients nowadays undergo further imaging with CT or MRI for better characterization of the coalition and preoperative planning.

Computed Tomography

CT scanning remains the standard imaging technique to demonstrate and evaluate tarsal coalition. Herzenberg and colleagues[59] used coronal CT images to evaluate tarsal coalitions in cadaveric specimens. They showed that CT demonstrated osseous and nonosseous coalitions in 14 of 22 specimens; in the remaining 8 specimens, CT effectively ruled out the diagnosis of subtalar coalition. They concluded that CT was superior to other modalities in identifying all aspects of the subtalar joint and talocalcaneal coalitions. CT assessment requires axial and coronal views of the feet and ankles. Cross-sectional thickness of 3 mm or less is optimal. Findings that suggest a calcaneonavicular coalition are joint-space narrowing, reactive sclerosis, medial broadening of the anterior and dorsal calcaneus on axial views, and rounding of the lateral talus on coronal views. Coronal CT views are the most useful in assessing talocalcaneal coalitions. Findings may include an osseous bridge at the middle facet, irregular cortices, broadening of the sustentaculum tali, and the drunken waiter sign (**Fig. 6**). The dysplatic sustentaculum may be upturned or downturned (likened to the hand of a waiter having difficulty carrying his tray), thereby sloping the joint line so it is no longer parallel to the posterior facet.[28,56] The advent of high-speed spiral

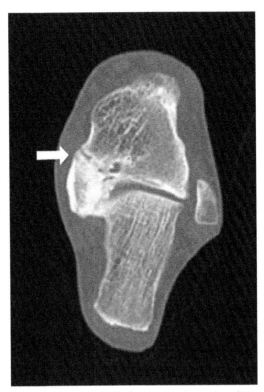

Fig. 6. Coronal CT image showing a middle-facet talocalcaneal coalition. Note the dysmorphic sustentaculum tali and upturned joint line (named the drunken waiter sign where the sustentaculum represents the hand and tray).

CT scanners and subsequent image reconstruction software has allowed good demonstration of talocalcaneal coalitions on coronal reconstructions of noncoronal CT views. CT is useful not only to confirm the diagnosis of coalition but also to define the size and location, assessing for degenerative changes such as subchondral sclerosis and cysts, and for preoperative planning. The radiation exposure for a CT scan of the foot is variable depending on the type of scanner and sequencing used. The approximate exposure dose is 2 to 4 mSv, which is comparable with the natural background radiation dose for 1 year.[60]

Magnetic Resonance Imaging

MRI scanning is advocated by some investigators for evaluating nonosseous coalitions and confirming the presence of arthrosis in the surrounding joints.[23,36,61] However, no good study has demonstrated significant diagnostic advantage over CT scanning. The protocol should ideally have 3 views of the feet and ankles: axial, coronal, and sagittal. Fat-suppressed sequences such as short-tau inversion recovery (STIR) or fat-suppressed T2-weighted sequences are useful in evaluating coalition in the presence of bone or soft-tissue edema. Osseous and ligamentous structures are evaluated using T1-/T2-weighted and fast spin-echo proton density–weighted images. As with CT imaging, sagittal and axial views are most useful in assessing calcaneonavicular coalitions and coronal views are best for talocalcaneal coalitions. A continuous bone marrow bridge may be seen in osseous coalitions, whereas articular narrowing and irregular joint cortices with marrow edema suggest a nonosseous coalition (**Fig. 7**). Nalaboff and Schweitzer[25] suggested that more subtle signs such as the reverse anteater and drunken waiter signs are better visualized on MRI. The high sensitivity of MRI is favored when a fibrous tarsal coalition is suspected, whereas CT is the standard imaging modality for detecting an osseous coalition and is more cost-effective.[30]

Nuclear Imaging

Bone scintigraphy has been proposed as a screening tool for tarsal coalition.[62] In 1982, Deutsch and colleagues[54] evaluated conventional radiography, bone scintigraphy, and CT scanning for the radiological assessment of 3 cases of talocalcaneal coalition. They found CT scanning provided the best visualization of the coalition site. In addition to the lack of anatomic detail, interpretation of scintigraphy is made more difficult by epiphyseal uptake present in children and adolescents, the population in which tarsal coalitions most commonly occur. With the decreasing expense of CT scans and increasing resolution of advanced multiplanar reconstruction, the use of bone scintigraphy in tarsal coalition has diminished. However, single-photon emission tomography (SPECT) may yield important localizing information in complex cases when used in conjunction with CT registration.[54,63]

TREATMENT

Treatment of symptomatic patients depends on the location and extent of the tarsal coalition, the severity of symptoms and the presence of degenerative changes. The

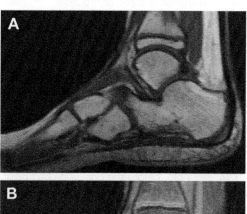
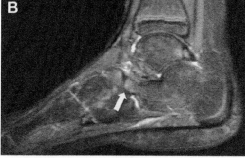

Fig. 7. (*A*) Sagittal MRI showing a calcaneonavicular coalition on T1-weighted image. (*B*) T2-weighted image of the same coalition with associated marrow edema (*arrow*).

patient's age, skeletal maturity and level of functional activity are important factors to take into account when considering operative treatment.

Nonoperative Treatment

Nonoperative therapy is usually the first line of treatment of symptomatic talocalcaneal and talonavicular coalitions.[11,23,49,64,65] This includes decreased activity, functional orthosis (ie, medial hindfoot wedge and arch support), antiinflammatory medication and University of California Berkeley Laboratory (UCBL) orthoses to prevent deterioration of the deformity in mildly symptomatic patients. If these simple measures fail to give pain relief, a limited period of immobilization in a cast or walker boot for 3 to 6 weeks may help. Cast immobilization decreases hindfoot and midfoot motion, reduces abnormal joint stresses and allows microfractures to heal. If symptoms settle after immobilization then physical therapy and a gradual return to full activities in a supportive shoe can be considered. These conservative measures can produce good results in cases of first presentation with no evidence of degenerative changes.[11,23,64,65]

Initial treatment of calcaneonavicular coalitions may include soft shoe inserts or a trial of walking-cast immobilization with the hindfoot in neutral if possible. It is reasonable to consider a second trial of cast immobilization if symptoms recur or persist, before conservative treatment is deemed unsuccessful. However, given the ease and relatively good results with surgical treatment, early resection of symptomatic calcaneonavicular coalitions in the younger patients have produced favorable results.[23,66,67]

Operative Treatment

Surgery is indicated in cases where conservative measures have failed to alleviate symptoms. The surgical options for tarsal coalition are resection or arthrodesis. Despite early studies recommending triple arthrodesis,[49,68] resection seems to be the appropriate treatment of calcaneonavicular coalitions, especially in the younger patients. The technique, as originally described by Badgley,[10] includes an anterolateral approach over the coalition, resection of at least 1 cm of the coalition, resecting a block rather than a wedge, interposition with the head of the extensor digitorum brevis (EDB) muscle, and avoid breaching the talonavicular capsule to prevent theoretical subluxation of the navicular over the talar head. Modifications of the original technique include use of bone wax after coalition resection and tying the interposition sutures over the plantar fascia, rather than securing them with a button over the plantar skin. Several long-term studies have shown 77% to 100% good or excellent results after calcaneonavicular coalition resection.[42,67,69] Cowell[14] suggested that the best outcome from resection of calcaneonavicular coalitions occurred when performed on patients less than 14 years old, before the coalitions had ossified. Routine use of an interpositional graft is necessary to reduce the recurrence of the coalition. Moyes and colleagues[70] performed a retrospective review of 17 calcaneonavicular coalition resections, of which 10 had EDB interposition and 7 had no soft-tissue interposition. Three in the second group had recurrence of the coalition along with their symptoms. Evidence for the ideal interposition graft remains controversial. The options include EDB muscle, bone wax, or fat. Cohen and colleagues[71] reported wound dehiscence in 3 out of 6 adult patients who underwent EDB transfer and bone wax application. Application of bone wax and gel foam produced similar results to those with EDB transfer, but with less wound complications. However, most studies in the pediatric population have reported good results using EDB interpositional grafts.

The optimal surgical management of symptomatic talocalcaneal coalitions has not been conclusively determined. Multiple factors have been described as important in predicting outcome including the patient's age, extent of the joint involved, degree of hindfoot valgus, and the presence of degenerative changes.[23] Before the advent of CT scanning, resection of the middle-facet talocalcaneal coalitions had unsatisfactory results because of poor preoperative visualization.[47] Hence, the surgical treatment of symptomatic talocalcaneal coalitions was traditionally a triple arthrodesis.[50,72] More recently, resections have become more popular and are indicated in cases in which conservative treatment has failed, CT/MRI visualization of the middle-facet coalition is good, and no degenerative changes are present in the posterior facet.[30] The surgical resection is approached medially, distal to the medial malleolus. The middle facet is exposed by retraction of the flexor hallucis longus (FHL) tendon inferiorly. The prominent joint is resected and interposition with either fat, split FHL tendon, or bone wax is performed.[73] To correct the residual valgus deformity, Luhmann and Schoenecker[52] recommended either a medializing calcaneal osteotomy if subtalar motion is restricted after coalition resection, otherwise, a lateral column lengthening. Giannini and colleagues[74] reported good or excellent hindfoot correction and pain relief in 11 out of 14 feet undergoing talocalcaneal coalition resection with correction of residual valgus using a bioabsorbable subtalar arthroereisis implant. Like Cowell,[14] they also recommended that patients younger than 14 years had better prognosis.

Comfort and Johnson[75] found a 77% success rate with resection when the coalition involved one-third or less of the total surface area of the subtalar joint on CT. Wilde and colleagues[76] found that a hindfoot valgus of greater than 16° and a coalition surface area greater than 50% of the posterior facet on CT were predictors of poor results after resection. Luhmann and Shoenecker[52] found that although an association existed between poor results and a heel valgus of more than 21° or a coalition greater than 50% of the posterior facet, some patients still had good postoperative results. They recommended that resection be tried initially, and the patient be counseled that they could still have a good result despite the presence of poor predictive factors. Long-term studies have shown variable good or excellent rates of 50% to 94% with resection of talocalcaneal coalition.[73,76,77] For cases in which a resection is not possible or desired, Mann and Baumgarten[78] proposed isolated fusion of the subtalar joint, instead of the traditional triple arthrodesis. Their reasoning was that any motion saved in the midtarsal joints would maintain force transfer during motion, decreasing any degenerative process in the adjacent joints. However, where degenerative changes in the midfoot are apparent, triple arthrodesis is indicated, as an isolated subtalar fusion would only accelerate the degenerative process. The presence of talar beaking seems to have no correlation to the outcome of coalition resection.[67,71,76] In 1983, Swiontkowski and colleagues[47] found no degenerative changes in the talonavicular joint on intraoperative inspection during resection of the talar beak. Therefore, isolated talar beaking is not a contraindication for resection surgery as it is not part of the degenerative change.

Salvage Surgery

Patients with unsuccessful excision of calcaneonavicular or talocalcaneal coalition have persistent pain. This may be attributed to incomplete resection, recurrent bone formation, or an ongoing degenerative process in the surrounding joints. Although some success has been reported with isolated subtalar fusion in small case series,[47,71] triple arthrodesis is the most reliable salvage procedure for failed resection surgery.

POSTOPERATIVE MANAGEMENT

The postoperative rehabilitation for resection surgery includes immobilization for 3 weeks in a non–weight-bearing cast, followed by partial immobilization in

a weight-bearing walker boot with range-of-motion exercises.[30] Postoperative rehabilitation for arthrodesis surgery involves immobilization for 3 weeks in a non–
weight-bearing cast, followed by 3 weeks of partial immobilization with a
non–weight-bearing walker boot with range-of-motion exercises out of the boot.
This is followed by a gradual advance to full weight bearing and range-of-motion exercises with physical therapy. Bilateral procedures are staged to allow full recovery of
the first foot before surgery on the second.

COMPLICATIONS

Infection and wound breakdown are possible complications with surgical treatment.[30,71] If symptoms fail to resolve after resection of the coalition, the subsequent
arthrodesis may be significantly compromised by ongoing infection. During resection
of a calcaneonavicular bar, violation of the talonavicular capsule may result in subluxation of the navicular on the talus, causing abnormal motion in the midfoot and risk of
further pain and degenerative changes.

OUTCOME/PROGNOSIS

Nonoperative treatment of patients with symptomatic tarsal coalitions has not been
uniformly successful and proper patient selection is a prerequisite for optimal results.
Patients with extensive or multiple coalitions typically undergo fusion procedures, and
those with less extensive or isolated coalitions undergo resection with soft-tissue
interposition. Most calcaneonavicular coalitions can be excised with the expectation
of successful long-term results. Resection of symptomatic talocalcaneal coalitions
yields optimal results when the coalition involves approximately one-third to half of
the posterior subtalar joint surface. The amount of postoperative subtalar movement
correlates well with clinical outcome.[42] Although there is no consensus regarding
patient's age as a predictor of success in coalition resection, it is reasonable to say
that some degenerative change is inevitably present at the time of presentation,[49]
especially in the older adolescents and adult cohort. Therefore, age may well be
a significant factor in predicting successful outcome for coalition resection, with
younger patients showing better prognosis.[49,66,74]

SUMMARY

Tarsal coalition is a relatively rare abnormality of the foot in which 2 or more of the
tarsal bones are joined by bone, cartilage, or fibrous tissue. Tarsal coalition is believed
to be a failure of mesenchymal differentiation and has an autosomal dominant inheritance with high penetrance. The incidence of symptomatic tarsal coalition is approximately 1%, but the true prevalence is unknown as most are asymptomatic.
Calcaneonavicular and talocalcaneal coalitions are the most common types. More
than half of tarsal coalitions are bilateral. Typically, the patient presents with a history
of chronic pain with activity, following a traumatic injury, or with repetitive sprains. Pain
from a tarsal coalition is believed to be generated by microfractures at the coalition-
bone interface. The condition is poorly visualized with conventional radiography, but
axial and 45° lateral oblique views offer better visualization. However, CT scanning
with coronal cuts is the gold standard investigation, particularly in evaluating talocalcaneal coalitions.
   Conservative treatment includes a medial heel wedge, arch support, and walking-
cast immobilization for 3 to 6 weeks. Surgical treatments for coalitions unresponsive to conservative measures include resection or arthrodesis. Calcaneonavicular

coalitions respond well to resection with interpositional graft, most commonly, EDB muscle belly. Currently, the true indications for resection of talocalcaneal coalitions have not been determined. Factors including heel valgus angle, patient age, and percentage of joint involvement do not produce consistent outcomes. Talar beaking does not indicate an arthritic joint and should not be a contraindication to resection. However, once global degenerative changes have begun, arthrodesis is the preferred surgical option. Routine use of CT and MRI is recommended to help make this decision. Subtalar arthrodesis is not sufficient in cases of talocalcaneal coalition where the midfoot joints are degenerate. It is also unproven as a salvage procedure for failed excision of a coalition. Triple arthrodesis is indicated in both circumstances.

REFERENCES

1. Coe WR, Broman VL. Tikal report no. 2. Excavations in the Stela 23 group. In Tikal reports nos. 1–4:23–60. University of Pennsylvania Museum Monograph No.15; 1958.
2. Heiple KG, Lovejoy CO. The antiquity of tarsal coalition: bilateral deformity in a pre-Columbian Indian skeleton. J Bone Joint Surg Am 1969;51:979–83.
3. Silva AM. Non-osseous calcaneonavicular coalition in the Portuguese prehistoric population: report of two cases. Int J Osteoarchaeol 2005;15:449–53.
4. Buffon GLL, Comte de. Histoire naturelle, générale et particulière, Tome 3. Paris: Imprimerie Royale; 1769. p. 47.
5. Cruveilhier J. Anatomie pathologique du corps humain. Tome 1. Paris: J B Baillière; 1829.
6. Zuckerkandl E. Ueber einen Fall von Synostose zwischen Talus und Calcaneus. Allgemeine Weiner Medizinische Zeitung 1877;22:293–4 [in German].
7. Anderson RJ. The presence of an astragalo-scaphoid bone in man. J Anat Physiol 1880;14(4):452–5.
8. Holl M. Beitrage zur chirurgischen osteologie des fusses. Langenbecks Arch Klin Chir 1880;25:211–23 [in German].
9. Slomann HC. On coalition calcaneo-navicularis. J Orthop Surg 1921;3: 586–602.
10. Badgley CE. Coalition of the calcaneus and the navicular. Arch Surg 1927;15: 75–88.
11. Harris RI, Beath T. Etiology of peroneal spastic flat foot. J Bone Joint Surg Br 1948;30:624–34.
12. Kirmisson E. Double pied bot varus par malformation osseuse primitive associe a des ankyloses congenitales des doigts et des arteils chez quatre membres di' une meme Famille. Revue d'Orthopedie 1898;9:392–8 [in French].
13. Korvin H. Coalitio Talocalcanea. Zeitschrift fuer Orthopaedische Chirurgie 1934; 60:105–10 [in German].
14. Cowell HR. Talocalcaneal coalition and new causes of peroneal spastic flatfoot. Clin Orthop 1972;85:16–22.
15. Mosier KM, Asher M. Tarsal coalitions and peroneal spastic flatfoot: a review. J Bone Joint Surg Am 1984;66:976–84.
16. Holland CT. Two cases of rare deformity of feet and hands. Archives of Radiology and Electrotherapy 1918;22:234–9.
17. Waugh W. Partial cubo-navicular coalition as a cause of peroneal spastic flat foot. J Bone Joint Surg Br 1957;39:520–3.
18. Lusby HLJ. Naviculo-cuneiform synostosis. J Bone Joint Surg Br 1959;41:150.

19. Wheeler R, Guevera A, Bleck EE. Tarsal coalitions: review of the literature and case report of bilateral dual calcaneonavicular and talocalcaneal coalitions. Clin Orthop Relat Res 1981;156:175–7.

20. Clarke DM. Multiple tarsal coalitions in the same foot. J Pediatr Orthop 1997;17: 777–80.

21. Stormont DM, Peterson HA. The relative incidence of tarsal coalition. Clin Orthop Relat Res 1983;181:28–36.

22. Kulik SA Jr, Clanton TO. Tarsal coalition. Foot Ankle Int 1996;17(5):286–96.

23. Lemley F, Berlet G, Hill K, et al. Current concepts review: tarsal coalition. Foot Ankle Int 2006;27(12):1163–9.

24. Rühl FJ, Solomon LB, Henneberg M. High prevalence of tarsal coalitions and tarsal joints variants in a recent cadaver sample and its possible significance. Clin Anat 2003;16(5):411–5.

25. Nalaboff KM, Schweitzer ME. MRI of tarsal coalition: frequency, distribution and innovative signs. Bull NYU Hosp Jt Dis 2008;66(1):14–21.

26. Lysack JT, Fenton PV. Variations in calcaneonavicular morphology demonstrated with radiography. Radiology 2004;230:493–7.

27. Soloman LB, Rühli FJ, Taylor J, et al. A dissection and computer tomography study of tarsal coalitions in 100 cadaver feet. J Orthop Res 2003;21:352–8.

28. Newman JS, Newberg AH. Congenital tarsal coalition: multimodality evaluation with emphasis on CT and MR imaging. Radiographics 2000;20(2):321–32.

29. Bohne WH. Tarsal coalition. Curr Opin Pediatr Feb 2001;13(1):29–35.

30. Vu L, Mehlman CT. Tarsal coalition. Updated Nov 2, 2007. eMedicine Specialities > Orthopaedic Surgery > Foot & Ankle (Medscape). Available at: http://emedicine. medscape.com/article/1233780-overview. Accessed August 13, 2009.

31. Leonard MA. The inheritance of tarsal coalition and its relationship to spastic flat foot. J Bone Joint Surg Br 1974;56(3):520–6.

32. Miki T, Yamamuro T, Iida H, et al. Naviculo-cuneiform coalition: a report of two cases. Clin Orthop 1985;196:256–9.

33. Kumai T, Tanaka Y, Takakura Y, et al. Isolated first naviculo-cuneiform joint coalition. Foot Ankle Int 1996;17:635–40.

34. Sato K, Sugiura S. Naviculo-cuneiform coalition – report of three cases [abstract]. Nippon Seikeigeka Gakkai Zasshi 1990;64(1):1–6.

35. Burnett SE, Case DT. Naviculo-cuneiform coalition: evidence of significant differences in tarsal coalition frequency. Foot 2005;15(2):80–5.

36. Wang EA, Gentili A, Masih S, et al. Tarsal coalition. Updated Jan 10, 2008. eMedicine Specialities > Radiology > Musculoskeletal (Medscape). Available at: http:// emedicine.medscape.com/article/396694-overview. Accessed August 13, 2009.

37. Harris BJ. Anomalous structures in the developing human foot. Anat Rec 1955; 121:399.

38. Leboucq H. De la soudure congenitale de certains os du tarse. Bull Acad R Méd Belg 1890;4:103–12 [in French].

39. Heikel HVA. Coalitio calcaneo-navicularis and calcaneus secundarius. A clinical and radiographic study of twenty-three patients. Acta Orthop Scand 1962;32: 72–84.

40. Wray JB, Herndon CN. Hereditary transmission of congenital coalition of the calcaneus to the navicular. J Bone Joint Surg Am 1963;45:365–72.

41. Pfitzner W. Die Variationen im Aufbau des Fusskelets. Morphologisches Arbeiten 1896;6:245–527 [in German].

42. Chambers RB, Cook TM, Cowell HR. Surgical reconstruction for calcaneonavicular coalition. J Bone Joint Surg Am 1982;64:829–36.

43. Plotkin S. Case presentation of calcaneonavicular coalition in monozygotic twins. J Am Podiatr Med Assoc 1996;86(9):433–8.
44. Manter JT. Movements of the subtalar and transverse tarsal joints. Anat Rec 1941; 80:397–410.
45. Wright DG, Desai SM, Henderson WH. Action of the subtalar and ankle-joint complex during the stance phase of walking. J Bone Joint Surg Am 1964;46:361–82.
46. Outland T, Murphy ID. The pathomechanics of peroneal spastic flat foot. Clin Orthop 1960;16:64–73.
47. Swiontkowski MF, Scranton PE, Hansen S. Tarsal coalitions: long-term results of surgical treatment. J Pediatr Orthop 1983;3:287–92.
48. Katayama T, Tanaka Y, Kadono K, et al. Talocalcaneal coalition: a case showing the ossification process. Foot Ankle Int 2005;26:490–3.
49. Cowell HR, Elener V. Rigid painful flatfoot secondary to tarsal coalition. Clin Orthop 1983;177:54–60.
50. Jayakumar S, Cowell HR. Rigid flatfoot. Clin Orthop 1977;122:77–84.
51. Kumai T, Takakura Y, Akiyama K, et al. Histopathological study of nonosseous tarsal coalitions. Foot Ankle Int 1998;19:525–31.
52. Luhmann SJ, Schoenecker PL. Symptomatic talocalcaneal coalition resection: indications and results. J Pediatr Orthop 1998;18(6):748–54.
53. Stuecker RD, Bennett JT. Tarsal coalition presenting as a pes cavo-varus deformity: report of three cases and review of the literature. Foot Ankle 1993;14: 540–4.
54. Deutsch AL, Resnick D, Campbell G. Computed tomography and bone scintigraphy in the evaluation of tarsal coalition. Radiology 1982;144:137–40.
55. Crim J, Kjeldsberg K. Radiographic diagnosis of tarsal coalition. Am J Roentgenol 2004;18:323–8.
56. Lateur LM. Subtalar coalition: diagnosis with the C sign on lateral radiographs of the ankle. Radiology 1994;193(3):847–51.
57. Sakellariou A, Sallomi D, Janzen DL, et al. Talocalcaneal coalition. Diagnosis with the C-sign on lateral radiographs of the ankle. J Bone Joint Surg Br 2000;82(4): 574–8.
58. Brown RR, Rosenberg ZS, Thornhill BA. The C sign: more specific for flatfoot deformity than subtalar coalition. Skeletal Radiol 2001;30(2):84–7.
59. Herzenberg JE, Goldner JL, Martinez S, et al. Computerized tomography of talocalcaneal tarsal coalition: a clinical and anatomic study. Foot Ankle 1986;6:273–88.
60. Radiation exposure from medical diagnostic procedures. Health Physics Society Fact Sheet. Available at: http://www.hps.org/documents/meddiagimaging.pdf. Accessed January 24, 2010.
61. Wechsler RJ, Schweitzer ME, Deely DM, et al. Tarsal coalition: depiction and characterization with CT and MR imaging. Radiology 1994;193:447–52.
62. Goldman AB, Pavlov H, Schneider R. Radionuclide bone scanning in subtalar coalitions: differential considerations. Am J Roentgenol 1982;138(3):427–32.
63. El Rassi G, Riddle EC, Kumar SJ. Arthrofibrosis involving the middle facet of the talocalcaneal joint in children and adolescents. J Bone Joint Surg Am 2005;87: 2227–31.
64. Morgan RC Jr, Crawford AH. Surgical management of tarsal coalition in adolescent athletes. Foot Ankle 1986;7:183–93.
65. Varner KE, Michelson JD. Tarsal coalition in adults. Foot Ankle Int 2000;21: 669–72.
66. Mitchell GP, Gibson JMC. Excision of calcaneo-navicular bar for painful spasmodic flat foot. J Bone Joint Surg Br 1967;49(2):281–7.

67. Gonzalez P, Kumar SJ. Calcaneonavicular coalition treated by resection and interposition of the extensor digitorum brevis muscle. J Bone Joint Surg Am 1990;72:71–7.
68. Andreason E. Calcaneo-navicular coalition: late results of resection. Acta Orthop Scand 1968;39:424–32.
69. Cowell HR. Extensor brevis arthroplasty. J Bone Joint Surg Am 1970;52:820.
70. Moyes ST, Crawfurd EJP, Aichroth PM. The interposition of extensor digitorum brevis in the resection of calcaneonavicular bars. J Pediatr Orthop 1994;14: 387–8.
71. Cohen BE, Davis WH, Anderson RB. Success of calcaneonavicular coalition resection in the adult population. Foot Ankle Int 1996;17:569–72.
72. Ehrlich MG, Elmer EB. Tarsal coalition. In: Jahss MH, editor. Disorders of the foot and ankle. 2nd edition. Philadelphia: WB Saunders; 1991. p. 921–8.
73. Kumar MD, Guille JT, Lee MS, et al. Osseous and non-osseous coalition of the middle facet of the talocalcaneal joint. J Bone Joint Surg Am 1992;74:529–35.
74. Giannini S, Ceccarelli F, Vannini F, et al. Operative treatment of flatfoot with talo-calcaneal coalition. Clin Orthop 2003;411:178–87.
75. Comfort TK, Johnson LO. Resection for symptomatic talocalcaneal coalition. J Pediatr Orthop 1998;18(3):283–8.
76. Wilde PH, Torode IP, Dickens DR, et al. Resection for symptomatic talocalcaneal coalition. J Bone Joint Surg Br 1994;76(5):797–801.
77. Takakura Y, Sugimoto K, Tanaka Y, et al. Symptomatic talocalcaneal coalition. Clin Orthop 1991;269:249–56.
78. Mann RA, Baumgarten M. Subtalar fusion for isolated subtalar disorders: preliminary report. Clin Orthop 1988;226:260–5.

The Use of Gait Analysis in the Treatment of Pediatric Foot and Ankle Disorders

Tim Theologis, MD, MSc, PhD, FRCS[a],*,
Julie Stebbins, DPhil, SRCS, CSci, MIPEM[b]

KEYWORDS
• Pediatric foot conditions • Gait analysis
• Dynamic foot assessment

DYNAMIC ASSESSMENT OF FOOT MOTION

Clinical assessment of ankle and foot problems in children is routinely based on relevant medical and family history, clinical examination, and imaging. Clinical assessment of the foot includes observation of the foot during standing, walking, or in performing various tasks, such as standing on tiptoes.

Dynamic assessment of ankle and foot motion during walking or other activities can offer valuable information but is challenging, particularly in young children. Observation during walking can provide only limited information on foot motion. For example, a child may display a foot drop, that is, plantarflexion of the foot during the swing phase of gait. Simple observation will not reveal if plantarflexion occurs at the ankle joint, at the midfoot joints, or both. This information is important when considering management decisions. If plantarflexion occurs at the ankle joint only and the forefoot remains well aligned in relation to the heel in a child with hemiplegia, for example, spasticity of the plantaflexors would be the likely cause of the problem. Detecting changes of foot shape and alignment between the stance and swing phases of gait can also offer valuable information that can influence decision making. Using simple

Disclosure statement: No funding support was received by any of the authors for the preparation of this article.
[a] Nuffield Orthopaedic Centre, Windmill Road, Headington, Oxford, OX3 7LD, UK
[b] Oxford Gait Laboratory, Nuffield Orthopaedic Centre, Windmill Road, Headington, Oxford, OX3 7LD, UK
* Corresponding author.
E-mail address: theologis@doctors.org.uk

Foot Ankle Clin N Am 15 (2010) 365–382
doi:10.1016/j.fcl.2010.02.002
1083-7515/10/$ – see front matter © 2010 Elsevier Inc. All rights reserved.

foot.theclinics.com

observation to obtain reliable information on relative motion between the anatomic segments of the foot during walking is a difficult task, because of the relatively small size of the foot, the speed with which changes occur, and the relatively small range of motion of foot joints. Furthermore, it is not possible to assess motion through palpation of anatomic landmarks during walking.

Video recordings of the feet during walking can offer additional information, compared with simple observation. Videos can be repeated to allow a more thorough observation and can offer recordings from different angles. Slow motion recordings can also contribute to a more thorough assessment. Changes in the shape and alignment of the foot can be further appreciated and the timing of these changes during the gait cycle can be identified. Activity of individual tendons can also be identified through close-up video recording and can offer valuable information on potential causes of a dynamic deformity. For example, the tibialis anterior tendon can be prominent and visible during the swing phase of gait in a hemiplegic child, which may imply that inappropriate activity of the tibialis anterior muscle is responsible for dynamic supination of the foot during the swing phase of gait. Despite these advantages over simple clinical observation, video recording as a method of assessing dynamic motion of the foot has significant limitations. Assessment of motion between anatomic segments of the foot is not quantifiable on video. Assessing the three-dimensional motion of relatively small anatomic structures on the two-dimensional video display is challenging, particularly in the presence of deformity and/or when recordings are not made in the same plane as the anatomic axes of the foot. Inaccurate and misleading interpretation can result.

Three-dimensional instrumented gait and motion analysis (3DGA) was initially introduced to allow detailed assessment and quantification of the motion of anatomic body segments during walking or other activities. Gait analysis was clinically established first in the management of ambulant children with cerebral palsy. Complex walking patterns and interactions between joints and muscles in this population are difficult to assess visually or with two-dimensional video. This situation, along with the need to assist clinical decisions before single-stage multilevel orthopedic surgery, led to the wide use of gait analysis.[1] The use of gait analysis has since expanded to include other neuromuscular conditions as well as orthopedic conditions in which complex gait patterns are difficult to assess clinically only.[2–4] 3DGA has been used extensively for clinical research in a variety of conditions affecting gait and for joint replacement design and outcome.[5,6] It is logical to expect that objective and quantifiable assessment of gait should be undertaken before and after treatment that sets gait improvement as one of its aims.

Instrumented gait analysis involves a multifaceted assessment tailored to the individual patient and the information required to assist clinical decisions. History and clinical examination form an integral part of the assessment and video recordings are always included. Kinematic analysis involves the study of motion of body segments and is usually displayed in graphs showing the motion of joints during the gait cycle. Combining this information with measurements from a force plate can provide the kinetic analysis, that is, the calculated moments, work, and power at each joint. Dynamic electromyography (EMG) can offer information about the timing of muscle activity during the gait cycle. The measurement of temporal and spatial parameters of gait, such as speed, cadence, step and stride length, and time, can offer further information about the overall quality and symmetry of gait. Energy consumption measurements also offer information on the quality and prognosis of walking. Plantar pressure measurements or dynamic pedobarography can provide information about the distribution of pressures under the foot at any given time of the gait cycle.

Conventional gait analysis usually represents the foot as a rigid body or a single vector and considers motion between this vector and the tibia only (**Fig. 1**). In the presence of significant foot deformity, this oversimplification can lead to significant error. In a planovalgus foot with significant midfoot break, for example, the forefoot may dorsiflex in relation to the tibia during late stance, while the hindfoot remains in equinus. For this reason, most gait analysis experts used to rely significantly on information from the video recordings to assess dynamic foot function, accepting the limitations as stated earlier. Secondary conclusions about the dynamic function of the foot were drawn from electromyographic and kinetic information. In recent years, however, the progress in motion analysis technology has offered higher resolution and

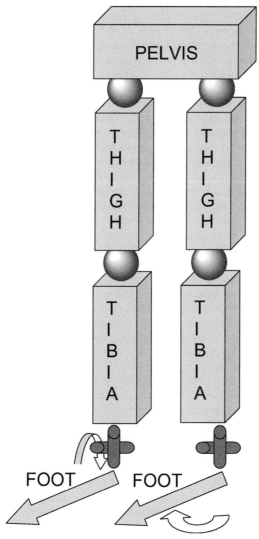

Fig. 1. The conventional lower body gait model. The pelvis, thighs, and tibiae are represented as three-dimensional segments with three-dimensional relative motion between them. The feet are represented as line vectors only.

increased precision in data acquisition, and has allowed clinicians and scientists to explore the analysis of relative motion between the anatomic segments of the foot during gait.

THE DEVELOPMENT OF KINEMATIC FOOT MODELS

In the initial years after the inception of clinical gait analysis, there were only a few centers involved in its practice and development. One standard model for representing human gait was proposed and almost unanimously accepted. This model is now variously referred to as the Newington, Davis, PlugInGait, or Conventional Model, but all these terms represent the same principle.[7] Because motion capture technology was also limited at the time, there was inherent restriction in the complexity of the model. Within this model, the foot was necessarily modeled in a simplistic manner. In conventional gait analysis, the motion of the pelvis, thighs, and lower legs are described in terms of three-dimensional movement of the distal segment in relation to the proximal segment, with the pelvis described in relation to an external reference frame (absolute vertical and horizontal). The feet, however, are represented as vectors only (see **Fig. 1**).[7]

The foot is a complex biomechanical structure composed of 28 bones and 33 joints. Unlike the more proximal segments of the lower body, it clearly does not behave as a rigid structure. Multisegment and multiplanar information is needed to accurately depict foot motion during gait. Multisegment foot models provide information about motion of the joints within the foot and at the ankle, by dividing the foot into 2 or more segments. Measurement of multisegment foot kinematics is becoming increasingly common as motion analysis systems improve in resolution and speed of data capture and processing. Numerous research groups around the world have proposed multisegment foot models, a summary of which is given in **Table 1**. Since the initial gait model was proposed and implemented, clinical gait analysis has become accepted around the world. There are now an estimated 200 laboratories worldwide. In addition, several major companies produce motion capture systems, based on widely different technology. It seems unlikely that a general consensus will be reached in the foreseeable future regarding the optimal method to model the foot during gait, as occurred with the original lower body model. However, the variety of models now available offers the opportunity to tailor an assessment according to the information required.

It has long been recognized that representing the foot as a single line provides inadequate information for dynamic assessment, particularly in the presence of foot deformity. Cadaveric studies have confirmed the complexity of foot and ankle mechanics and the need for accurate models.[42,43] As far back as the late 1980s there were initial forays into multisegment foot modeling. Kepple and colleagues[8] were among the first to implement and publish an alternative model. They defined three-dimensional hindfoot (calcaneus) and lower leg (tibia) segments and tested their model on 5 healthy adult subjects. They proposed a similar convention for the calculation and output of angles as that used for the more proximal joints of the lower body. This resulted in motion that was described in 3 perpendicular planes.

In the early to mid-1990s, several other models were proposed. Scott and Winter,[9] Siegel and colleagues,[11] Moseley and colleagues,[20] and Liu and colleagues[21] all continued to develop 2-segment models composed of lower leg and hindfoot segments. The mathematical techniques for modeling the segments differed between investigators. In particular, there was disagreement as to whether the angles during gait should be referenced to a standard neutral position (usually subtalar neutral) or represented as actual angles. Referencing to a neutral standing position is feasible for the measurement of healthy feet, but it presents a challenge when studying pathologic feet, particularly when structural deformity is present. This question continues to be debated, with no clear consensus yet established.

By the late 1990s, multisegment foot models began to include 3 or more segments. In 1996, Kidder and colleagues[12] proposed a 4-segment model, which included the lower leg, hindfoot, forefoot, and hallux. This model is now referred to as the Milwaukee Foot Model. Several other models that have been published since then have included the same 4 segments, although they differ substantially in anatomic and mathematical descriptions of these segments.[10,22,29,30] Other variations of multisegment foot models have also been proposed. Hunt and colleagues[24] and Kitaoka and colleagues[36] suggested models that exclude the hallux, whereas Wu and colleagues[23] and Leardini and colleagues[26,27] included a midfoot segment in their models. Several models also separated the forefoot into medial and lateral segments, or considered the first metatarsal separately.[26,37–39,41] The model proposed by MacWilliams and colleagues[34] is composed of 9 distinct segments, including the lower leg, calcaneus, talus and navicular, cuboid, lateral forefoot, medial forefoot, lateral toes, medial toes, and hallux. One group has suggested a different approach to representing foot motion during gait. They suggested using two-dimensional angles rather than three-dimensional segment rotations.[35]

Most research to date has been conducted on healthy adult feet.[8–10,12,22–24,26,27,29,35–39,41] Only the Oxford Foot Model (OFM)[30,32] and MacWilliams and colleagues[34] have assessed motion of the foot in children. This population poses different challenges compared with measuring adult feet, the most significant being the small surface area of the foot, and greater variability of motion.[44] Most studies are also generally limited to the stance phase of the gait cycle. Only a few studies have assessed both stance and swing phases.[12,23,25,29,30,35,38] A growing number of studies have implemented multisegment foot models to assess patients with a variety of conditions leading to foot deformity but these have mainly been restricted to the adult population. The Milwaukee Foot Model has been applied to assess ankle arthrosis,[13] rheumatoid arthritis,[15] hallux rigidus,[16] and posterior tibialis tendon dysfunction.[17–19] Tome and colleagues[37] also measured subjects with posterior tibialis tendon dysfunction. Published studies using the OFM have included assessment of clubfoot,[5] forefoot varus,[33] and hemiplegic cerebral palsy.[31] Woodburn and colleagues[25] and Siegel and colleagues[11] have assessed rheumatoid arthritis. In addition, ankle arthrodesis,[23] midfoot arthritis,[40] diabetes,[39] and low-mobile feet[41] have been assessed by various investigators.

It is important that the reliability and clinical significance of these models be investigated thoroughly before their implementation in routine clinical practice. It is also necessary to standardize the analysis and the reporting of results.

THE OFM

The OFM was first proposed by Carson and colleagues[29] in 2001. The model is composed of a rigid lower leg segment (tibia and fibula), hindfoot segment (calcaneus), forefoot segment (5 metatarsals), and a hallux (**Fig. 2**). Markers are placed on 5 anatomic landmarks for each segment, which ensures enough markers are visible by the motion analysis cameras at any given stage of the gait cycle (**Fig. 3**).

The model was initially tested for reliability on 2 healthy adults[29] and has also been applied to children with talipes equinovarus[5] in evaluating residual clubfoot deformity. However, these measurements were restricted to the stance phase of the gait cycle. Modifications were then made to the original model to allow its application to children

Table 1
Multisegment foot models summary

Model	Model Description				Pathologic Studies				
	Segments	Gait Cycle	Subjects	References	Pathology	Subjects	Outcome	References
Kepple	Tibia Hindfoot	Stance	5 adults	Kepple et al (1990)[8]	NO	NA	NA	NA
Scott	Tibia Hindfoot	Stance	3 adults	Scott and Winter (1991)[9]	NO	NA	NA	NA
D'Andrea	Tibia Hindfoot Forefoot Hallux	Stance	1 subject	D'Andrea et al (1993)[10]	NO	NA	NA	NA
Siegel	Tibia Foot	Stance	1 adult control, 1 pronated foot	Siegel et al (1995)[11]	Rheumatoid arthritis	4 adults	Sensitivity to detect abnormality	Siegel et al (1995)[11]
Milwaukee Foot Model	Tibia Hindfoot Forefoot Hallux	Stance swing	1 adult Adults	Kidder et al (1996)[12] Myers et al (2004)[14]	Ankle arthrosis Rheumatoid arthritis Hallux rigidus PTTD PTTD PTTD	34 adults 22 adults 22 adults 34 adults 20 adults 20 adults	Define specific pathologic motion Define specific pathologic motion Define specific pathologic motion Define specific pathologic motion Effect of surgery Compare different types of treatment	Khazzam et al (2006)[13] Khazzam et al (2007)[15] Canseco et al (2008)[16] Ness et al (2008)[17] Brodsky et al (2009)[18] Marks et al (2009)[19]
Moseley	Tibia Hindfoot	Stance	14 adults	Moseley et al (1996)[20]	NO	NA	NA	NA
Liu	Tibia Hindfoot	Stance	10 adults	Liu et al (1997)[21]	NO	NA	NA	NA

Model	Segments	Phase	N	Reference	Condition	N	Purpose	Reference
Rattanaprasert	Tibia, Hindfoot, Forefoot, Hallux	Stance	10 adults	Rattanaprasert et al (1999)[22]	PTTD	1 adult	Sensitivity to detect abnormality	Rattanaprasert et al (1999)[22]
Wu	Tibia, Hindfoot/midfoot Forefoot	Stance Swing	10 adults	Wu et al (2000)[23]	Ankle arthrodesis	10 adults	Quantify pathologic motion	Wu et al. (2000)[23]
Hunt	Tibia, Hindfoot, Forefoot	Stance	18 adults	Hunt et al (2001)[24]	NO	NA	NA	NA
Woodburn	Tibia, Hindfoot	Stance Swing	?	Woodburn et al (2002)[25]	Rheumatoid arthritis	50 adults	Compare barefoot and shoes	Woodburn et al (2002)[25]
IOR version 1	Tibia, Hindfoot, Midfoot, First metatarsal, Hallux	Stance	9 adults	Leardini et al (1999)[26]	NO	NA	NA	NA
IOR version 2	Tibia, Foot, Hindfoot, Midfoot, Forefoot + 2D lines	Stance	10 adults	Leardini et al (2007)[27]	NO	NA	NA	NA
			3 adults	Chang et al (2008)[28]	NO	NA	NA	NA
Oxford Foot Model	Tibia, Hindfoot, Forefoot, Hallux vector	Stance Swing	2 adults	Carson et al (2001)[29]	Clubfoot	20 children	Quantify pathologic motion	Theologis et al (2003)[5]
			15 children	Stebbins et al (2006)[30]	CP hemiplegia	16 children	Assess repeatability of model	Stebbins et al (2008)[31]
			8 children	Curtis et al (2009)[32]	Forefoot varus	10 children, 11 controls	Assess compensation	Alonso-Vazquez et al (2009)[33]

(continued on next page)

Table 1
(continued)

Model	Model Description				Pathologic Studies			
	Segments	Gait Cycle	Subjects	References	Pathology	Subjects	Outcome	References
MacWilliams	Tibia Calcaneus Talus/navicular Cuboid Lateral forefoot Medial forefoot Lateral toes Medial toes Hallux	Stance	18 children	MacWilliams et al (2003)[34]	NA	NO	NO	NO
Heidelberg Foot Model	NA	Stance Swing	10 adults	Simon et al (2006)[35]	NA	NO	NO	NO
Kitaoka	Tibia Hindfoot Forefoot	Stance	20 adults	Kitaoka et al (2006)[36]	NA	NO	NO	NO
Tome	Tibia Hindfoot Medial forefoot Lateral forefoot Hallux	Stance	10 adults	Tome et al (2006)[37]	PTTD	14 adults	Compare differences with reference data	Tome et al (2006)[37]
Jenkyn	Hindfoot Midfoot Medial forefoot Lateral forefoot	Stance Swing	12 adults	Jenkyn & Nicol (2007)[38]	NA	NO	NO	NO
Rao/Wilken	Tibia Calcaneus First metatarsal Forefoot	Stance	15 adults	Rao et al (2007)[39]	Diabetes Midfoot arthritis	15 adults 30 adults	Compare differences with reference data Compare differences with referencedata	Rao et al (2007)[39] Rao et al (2009)[40]
Cobb	Hindfoot Midfoot Medial forefoot First metatarsal	Stance	11 adults	Cobb et al (2009)[41]	Low-mobile feet	11 adults	Compare differences with reference data	Cobb et al (2009)[41]

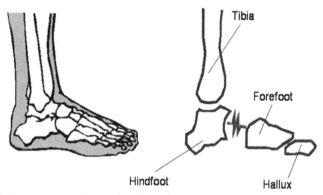

Fig. 2. The OFM consisting of tibia, hindfoot, forefoot, and optional hallux segments.

with foot deformity resulting from cerebral palsy. The specific aim was to accurately represent motion of the foot where significant deformity was present. For this to be practically feasible, the model needed to be easily applied within a clinical context, and provide meaningful results to clinicians.

Once the model had been adapted, it was discovered that the repeatability was diminished compared with the tests conducted on healthy adults. This was particularly evident in the transverse plane. To address this issue, 5 variations of the default model were tested for anatomic feasibility and repeatability. All 5 variations of the model were compared with the default model for repeatability. Based on this study, the model was finalized and has since been published.[30] To our knowledge, only the OFM has been assessed for repeatability in a pathologic population. Children with hemiplegic cerebral palsy were assessed on 3 separate occasions. The variability was found to be similar to typically developing children.[31]

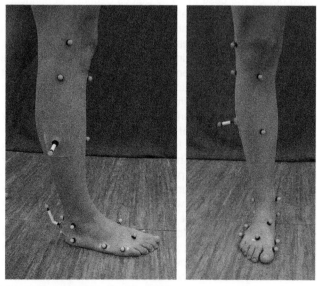

Fig. 3. Anatomic marker positions for the OFM.

Awareness of the variability in measurement of intersegment foot motion in children is vital for accurate interpretation of results and should not be ignored when planning treatment and assessing outcomes. Although several variations of the OFM were assessed for measuring foot motion, up to 7° of variability was still apparent in the transverse plane. It was recognized that this may be due in part to the inherent variability in children's gait. However, a significant factor is the consistency of marker placement between days on small feet. Therefore, clear protocols and practice in marker placement are crucial for achieving reliable results.

CLINICAL USE OF THE OFM

Our clinical experience in using the OFM amounts to approximately 400 patients, of which 40 have been assessed on more than 1 occasion. Two hundred of these patients were children with cerebral palsy and 40 were children with treated clubfeet. The remainder represented a variety of orthopedic and neuromuscular disorders. In half of these patients, dynamic assessment of foot motion significantly influenced the clinical decision making on their management. In those patients, the information obtained from the gait analysis and the OFM, in particular, was used to clarify the location of dynamic deformity (eg, internal rotation at hindfoot level compared with forefoot adduction), to clarify controversial findings from the clinical examination or conventional kinematics, to monitor progression of dynamic foot deformity over time, and to assess the outcome of treatment. The findings contributed to clinical decisions on surgical or orthotic management.

We use gait analysis when patients with cerebral palsy are being considered for surgical treatment, either in the form of multilevel surgery or simply for correction of foot deformity. We also use gait analysis in patients with cerebral palsy when there are unresolved questions about their conservative management (eg, physiotherapy, orthotics, botulinum toxin). In our institution we also follow up patients with cerebral palsy with gait analysis at 12 months postoperatively to assess the outcome. We realize this would not be the case in some places because of financial constraints. We found gait analysis particularly useful in patients with three-dimensional dynamic deformity of the foot (or the lower limb in general), as mentioned elsewhere in this article. In clubfoot patients, we found gait analysis useful only in a small group of older children (>5–6 years of age) who have impaired function or symptoms despite a satisfactory result. In some of these children, we found that dynamic problems can occur during gait but are not obvious on clinical examination. These problems can often explain their symptoms or functional limitations.

We studied 43 feet in diplegic patients with cerebral palsy and found consistently reduced sagittal motion of the hindfoot and the forefoot, as expected. In the coronal and transverse planes, however, we found a variety of deviations of foot motion, compared with our normal database. This implies that dynamic foot deformity in diplegic patients does not follow a uniform pattern and reinforces the need for an in-depth study of dynamic foot motion before any decisions on management are made.

In a study of 70 hemiplegic patients with cerebral palsy we also found limited range of motion of the hindfoot and forefoot in the sagittal plane, with limited dorsiflexion being the most prevalent problem. Most patients demonstrated internal rotation of the hindfoot combined with inversion, which reflects the prevalent equinovarus foot deformity in this patient population. However, there was still variation in the observed patterns and no uniformity in the findings across the whole population, which further reinforces the need to study dynamic motion of the foot in this population.

We used gait analysis in a prospective study to assess the outcome of foot surgery in hemiplegia.[45] We compared 12 hemiplegic patients with 14 age-matched controls and compared postoperative results at 6 and 12 months after treatment with the patients' preoperative findings. We used the OFM to analyze in detail the effects of surgery on the function of the foot pre- and postoperatively. Surgical treatment involved a combination of soft tissue and bone procedures, the choice of which depended on the preoperative clinical assessment and gait analysis findings. We found that hindfoot position and motion in the sagittal and coronal planes improved significantly. At the forefoot, adduction improved postoperatively but sagittal motion was variable and some patients showed increased plantarflexion at 12 months postoperatively. Plantar pressure distribution also improved after surgery. Conventional gait analysis demonstrated a series of improvements in proximal joints resulting from the correction of the foot deformity, including pelvic rotation, hip extension, and knee hyperextension. This study demonstrated in an objective way the outcome of foot surgery in this patient population.

In the early stages of development of the OFM, we undertook a study of patients with surgically treated clubfeet (before the introduction of the Ponseti technique in our unit) and a good or excellent result on the clinical and patient-derived outcome measures.[5] We demonstrated that, despite the perception of a satisfactory clinical result, significant gait deviations persisted. These included a tendency to hyperextend at knee level and to externally rotate at the hip. There was also reduced range of hindfoot motion, consistent with the postsurgical stiffness observed in these patients. This study offered an objective measure of dynamic performance of clubfeet with a satisfactory surgical outcome. We still use this information to objectively assess if patients with treated clubfeet who present with symptoms or functional problems perform within the limits defined by this study or display more severe deviations.

We have not analyzed a sufficient number of clubfeet treated with the Ponseti technique to draw any safe conclusions. This would imply of course that children treated with the Ponseti technique function well and are not referred often for gait analysis. Their feet are probably more flexible during walking that those of children treated surgically, but because of our small numbers, we have not yet been able to verify this.

More recently we undertook a study of 23 patients with clubfeet treated surgically to compare the findings of a standardized clinical examination of their feet to the findings of gait analysis and the OFM.[46] We found that in 16 of the 23 feet studied there was an element of deformity that was either only static or only dynamic but not both. For example, residual cavus observed on clinical examination was not always present during walking or dynamic forefoot supination was only present during walking. This comparison between static and dynamic foot deformity further illustrates the clinical application of gait analysis in the treatment of foot problems in children.

A short case study is presented to illustrate the use of motion analysis and the OFM in clinical decision making.

A 9-year-old male patient with right hemiplegia caused by cerebral palsy presented with a deteriorating gait and pain around his right ankle and foot. He maintained a high functional level, being able to walk 15 minutes to school and participate in sports and physical education using a right ankle foot orthosis. Clinical examination revealed cavovarus alignment of the foot on weight bearing but this was fully correctable passively. He also had 10° of fixed equinus deformity, a leg length discrepancy of 1.5 cm (right shorter), tight hamstrings on the right with a popliteal angle of 50° and a trace of fixed flexion deformity at the right hip.

His conventional lower limb gait analysis (**Fig. 4**) confirmed persistent foot plantarflexion on the right and an internal foot progression (intoeing) arising from the

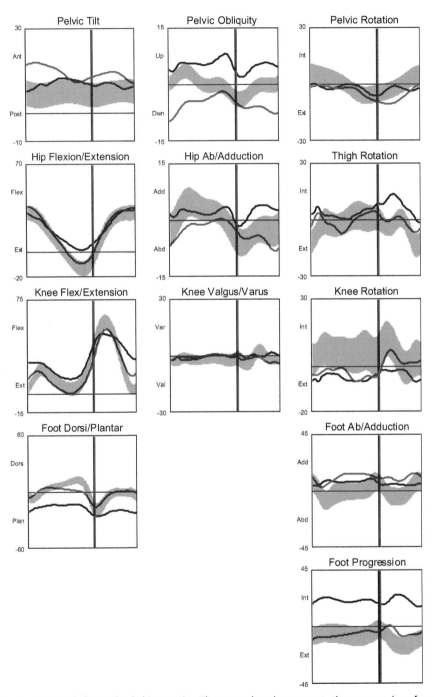

Fig. 4. Case study lower body kinematics. The green band represents the mean values from our normal database (±1SD). Red is from the left leg, and blue from the right leg. Each graph is normalized to a gait cycle.

deforrmity of the foot and internal tibial torsion. Foot kinematics using the OFM (**Fig. 5**) showed that there was plantarflexion of the hindfoot in relation to the tibia (plantarflexors' tightness/spasticity) but also of the forefoot in relation to the hindfoot (cavus). The OFM confirmed that forefoot adduction in relation to the hindfoot contributed to the intoeing gait. There was also an unusual combination of hindfoot inversion with forefoot supination. In the presence of hindfoot inversion in hemiplegia the forefoot usually

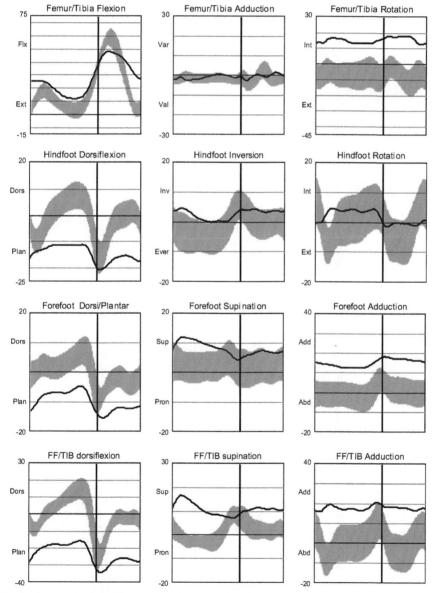

Fig. 5. Case study OFM kinematics. The green band represents the mean values from our normal database (±1SD). The blue line represents data from the right leg. Each graph is normalized to a gait cycle.

assumes a compensatory position of pronation during weight bearing in stance. The supination of the forefoot in this patient implied that there were different deforming forces acting on the hindfoot and the forefoot. We assumed that abnormal tibialis anterior activity was responsible for the forefoot adduction/supination and that spasticity and tightness of the gastrocnemius and tibialis posterior was causing the hindfoot varus.

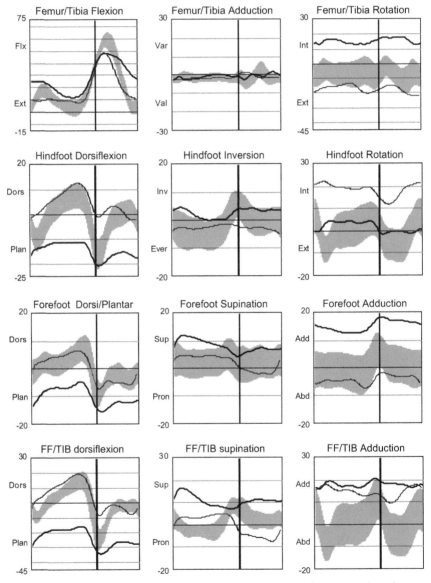

Fig. 6. Case study OFM kinematics. The green band represents the mean values from our normal database (±1SD). The thick blue line represents data from the right leg preoperatively. The thin blue line represents postoperative data. Each graph is normalized to a gait cycle.

From the clinical and gait analysis findings, surgical treatment was recommended, including lengthening of the gastrocnemius and tibialis posterior and a split tibialis anterior transfer. Six months postoperatively the foot deformity was well corrected in all 3 planes, on static and dynamic assessments (**Fig. 6**).

So far, the validation of multisegment foot models has mostly consisted of repeatability studies and comparison with data derived from cadaveric studies. More robust methods to determine reliability of these models is required. Recent studies have been based on metal pins inserted in the bone of the foot in vivo to quantify actual movement of each joint within the foot.[47–50] The results of these studies have added important information to the understanding of foot mechanics during walking. Further validation by comparison with data obtained from imaging techniques could improve the accuracy and reliability of these models. In addition, combination of foot kinematic modeling with other measurement modalities, such as imaging or plantar pressure assessment, may add more in-depth knowledge and understanding of how the foot behaves during gait. We are currently developing a method to combine the OFM with plantar pressure assessment,[51] with encouraging results.

We believe that assessment of foot pathology during walking should form an integral part of the clinical evaluation of children. Simple observation and video recording have limitations and are not quantifiable. Three-dimensional analysis of foot motion during walking can add invaluable information on the dynamic function of the foot and can contribute to clinical decision making. As motion analysis technology advances, the accuracy and reliability of the dynamic assessment of the foot during walking will increase further, allowing clinicians to rely confidently on this information during patient assessment and the study of treatment outcomes. As stated earlier, it is logical to expect that objective and quantifiable assessment of gait should be undertaken before and after treatment that sets gait improvement as one of its aims.

REFERENCES

1. Gage J, editor. The treatment of gait problems in cerebral palsy. London: Mac Keith Press; 2004.
2. Duffy CM, Hill AE, Cosgrove AP, et al. Three-dimensional gait analysis in spina bifida. J Pediatr Orthop 1996;16(6):786–91.
3. Westhoff B, Petermann A, Hirsch MA, et al. Computerized gait analysis in Legg Calve Perthes disease–analysis of the frontal plane. Gait Posture 2006;24(2): 196–202.
4. Karol LA, Halliday SE, Gourineni P. Gait and function after intra-articular arthrodesis of the hip in adolescents. J Bone Joint Surg Am 2000;82(4):561–9.
5. Theologis TN, Harrington ME, Thompson N, et al. Dynamic foot movement in children treated for congenital talipes equinovarus. J Bone Joint Surg Br 2003;85(4): 572–7.
6. Leardini A, O'Connor JJ, Catani F, et al. Mobility of the human ankle and the design of total ankle replacement. Clin Orthop Relat Res 2004;424:39–46.
7. Davis RB, Deluca PA. Clinical gait analysis. In: Harris GF, Smith P, editors. Human motion analysis. New Jersey (USA): IEEE Press; 1996. p. 17–42.
8. Kepple TM, Stanhope SJ, Lohmann KN, et al. A video-based technique for measuring ankle-subtalar motion during stance. J Biomed Eng 1990;12(4): 273–80.
9. Scott SH, Winter DA. Talocrural and talocalcaneal joint kinematics and kinetics during the stance phase of walking. J Biomech 1991;24(8):743–52.

10. D'Andrea S, Tylkowski C, Losito J, et al. Three-dimensional kinematics of the foot. Presented at the Eighth Annual East Coast Clinical Gait Conference. Rochester (MN), May 5–8, 1993.
11. Siegel KL, Kepple TM, O'Connell PG, et al. A technique to evaluate foot function during the stance phase of gait. Foot Ankle Int 1995;16(12):764–70.
12. Kidder SM, Abuzzahab FS Jr, Harris GF, et al. A system for the analysis of foot and ankle kinematics during gait. IEEE Trans Rehabil Eng 1996;4(1): 25–32.
13. Khazzam M, Long JT, Marks RM, et al. Preoperative gait characterization of patients with ankle arthrosis. Gait Posture 2006;24(1):85–93.
14. Myers KA, Wang M, Marks RM, et al. Validation of a multisegment foot and ankle kinematic model for pediatric gait. IEEE Trans Neural Syst Rehabil Eng 2004; 12(1):122–30.
15. Khazzam M, Long JT, Marks RM, et al. Kinematic changes of the foot and ankle in patients with systemic rheumatoid arthritis and forefoot deformity. J Orthop Res 2007;25(3):319–29.
16. Canseco K, Long J, Marks R, et al. Quantitative characterization of gait kinematics in patients with hallux rigidus using the Milwaukee Foot Model. J Orthop Res 2008;26(4):419–27.
17. Ness ME, Long J, Marks R, et al. Foot and ankle kinematics in patients with posterior tibial tendon dysfunction. Gait Posture 2008;27(2):331–9.
18. Brodsky JW, Charlick DA, Coleman SC, et al. Hindfoot motion following reconstruction for posterior tibial tendon dysfunction. Foot Ankle Int 2009;30(7): 613–8.
19. Marks RM, Long JT, Ness ME, et al. Surgical reconstruction of posterior tibial tendon dysfunction: prospective comparison of flexor digitorum longus substitution combined with lateral column lengthening or medial displacement calcaneal osteotomy. Gait Posture 2009;29(1):17–22.
20. Moseley L, Smith R, Hunt A, et al. Three-dimensional kinematics of the rearfoot during the stance phase of walking in normal young adult males. Clin Biomech (Bristol, Avon) 1996;11(1):39–45.
21. Liu W, Siegler S, Hillstrom HJ, et al. Three-dimensional, six-degrees-of-freedom kinematics of the human hindfoot during stance phase of level walking. Hum Mov Sci 1997;16:283–98.
22. Rattanaprasert U, Smith R, Sullivan M, et al. Three-dimensional kinematics of the forefoot, rearfoot, and leg without the function of tibialis posterior in comparison with normals during stance phase of walking. Clin Biomech (Bristol, Avon) 1999;14(1):14–23.
23. Wu WL, Su FC, Cheng YM, et al. Gait analysis after ankle arthrodesis. Gait Posture 2000;11(1):54–61.
24. Hunt AE, Smith RM, Torode M, et al. Inter-segment foot motion and ground reaction forces over the stance phase of walking. Clin Biomech (Bristol, Avon) 2001; 16(7):592–600.
25. Woodburn J, Helliwell PS, Barker S. Three-dimensional kinematics at the ankle joint complex in rheumatoid arthritis patients with painful valgus deformity of the rearfoot. Rheumatology (Oxford) 2002;41(12):1406–12.
26. Leardini A, Benedetti MG, Catani F, et al. An anatomically based protocol for the description of foot segment kinematics during gait. Clin Biomech (Bristol, Avon) 1999;14(8):528–36.
27. Leardini A, Benedetti MG, Berti L, et al. Rear-foot, mid-foot and fore-foot motion during the stance phase of gait. Gait Posture 2007;25(3):453–62.

28. Chang R, Van Emmerik R, Hamill J. Quantifying rearfoot-forefoot coordination in human walking. J Biomech 2008;4(14):3101–5.

29. Carson MC, Harrington ME, Thompson N, et al. Kinematic analysis of a multi-segment foot model for research and clinical applications: a repeatability analysis. J Biomech 2001;34(10):1299–307.

30. Stebbins J, Harrington M, Thompson N, et al. Repeatability of a model for measuring multi-segment foot kinematics in children. Gait Posture 2006;23(4): 401–10.

31. Stebbins J, Zavatsky A, Thompson N, et al. Repeatability of the Oxford Foot Model in hemiplegic cerebral palsy. Gait Posture 2008;28(Suppl 2):S21–2.

32. Curtis DJ, Bencke J, Stebbins JA, et al. Intra-rater repeatability of the Oxford foot model in healthy children in different stages of the foot roll over process during gait. Gait Posture 2009;30(1):118–21.

33. Alonso-Vazquez A, Villarroya MA, Franco MA, et al. Kinematic assessment of paediatric forefoot varus. Gait Posture 2009;29(2):214–9.

34. MacWilliams BA, Cowley M, Nicholson DE. Foot kinematics and kinetics during adolescent gait. Gait Posture 2003;17(3):214–24.

35. Simon J, Doederlein L, McIntosh AS, et al. The Heidelberg foot measurement method: development, description and assessment. Gait Posture 2006;23(4): 411–24.

36. Kitaoka HB, Crevoisier XM, Hansen D, et al. Foot and ankle kinematics and ground reaction forces during ambulation. Foot Ankle Int 2006;27(10):808–13.

37. Tome J, Nawoczenski DA, Flemister A, et al. Comparison of foot kinematics between subjects with posterior tibialis tendon dysfunction and healthy controls. J Orthop Sports Phys Ther 2006;36(9):635–44.

38. Jenkyn TR, Nicol AC. A multi-segment kinematic model of the foot with a novel definition of forefoot motion for use in clinical gait analysis during walking. J Biomech 2007;40(14):3271–8.

39. Rao S, Saltzman C, Yack HJ. Segmental foot mobility in individuals with and without diabetes and neuropathy. Clin Biomech (Bristol, Avon) 2007;22(4): 464–71.

40. Rao S, Baumhauer JF, Tome J, et al. Comparison of in vivo segmental foot motion during walking and step descent in patients with midfoot arthritis and matched asymptomatic control subjects. J Biomech 2009;42(8):1054–60.

41. Cobb SC, Tis LL, Johnson JT, et al. The effect of low-mobile foot posture on multi-segment medial foot model gait kinematics. Gait Posture 2009;30(3):334–9.

42. Engsberg JR. A biomechanical analysis of the talocalcaneal joint–in vitro. J Biomech 1987;20(4):429–42.

43. Siegler S, Chen J, Schneck CD. The three-dimensional kinematics and flexibility characteristics of the human ankle and subtalar joints–part I: kinematics. J Biomech Eng 1988;110(4):364–73.

44. Stolze H, Kuhtz-Buschbeck JP, Mondwurf C, et al. Retest reliability of spatiotemporal gait parameters in children and adults. Gait Posture 1998;7(2):125–30.

45. Stebbins JA. The identification and analysis of compensatory mechanisms in children with foot deformity resulting from cerebral palsy. Oxford: Nuffield Department of Orthopaedic Surgery, Oxford University; 2005.

46. McCahill J, Stebbins J, Theologis T. Comparison or residual deformity in clubfeet using a clinical exam and the Oxford foot model. Gait Posture 2008;28(Suppl 2): S43–4.

47. Arndt A, Wolf P, Liu A, et al. Intrinsic foot kinematics measured in vivo during the stance phase of slow running. J Biomech 2007;40(12):2672–8.

48. Lundgren P, Nester C, Liu A, et al. Invasive in vivo measurement of rear-, mid- and forefoot motion during walking. Gait Posture 2008;28(1):93–100.
49. Nester C, Jones RK, Liu A, et al. Foot kinematics during walking measured using bone and surface mounted markers. J Biomech 2007;40(15):3412–23.
50. Wolf P, Stacoff A, Liu A, et al. Functional units of the human foot. Gait Posture 2008;28(3):434–41.
51. Stebbins JA, Harrington ME, Giacomozzi C, et al. Assessment of sub-division of plantar pressure measurement in children. Gait Posture 2005;22(4):372–6.

Index

Note: Page numbers of article titles are in **boldface** type.

A

Accessory naviculars (ANs), **337–347**
    adolescent, **337–347**
    anatomy of, 337–338
    classification of, 338–339
    clinical presentation of, 339
    described, 337
    embryology of, 337–338
    imaging of, 339–341
    management of
        author's preferred treatment, 344–345
        conservative, 341–342
        surgical, 342–344
Adolescent(s), ANs in, **337–347**. See also Accessory naviculars (ANs).
Ankle deformities, severe, Ilizarov external fixation in correction of, **265–285**. See also
    Ilizarov external fixation, in correction of severe pediatric foot and ankle deformities, .
Ankle disorders. See Foot and ankle disorders; specific deformities/disorders and Foot and
    ankle deformities.
ANs. See Accessory naviculars (ANs).
Arthritis, as adult sequela of treated clubfoot, 294
Arthrodesis, triple, for clubfoot, 261
Arthroereisis, subtalar, in flatfoot reconstruction in children, **323–335**. See also Subtalar
    arthroereisis, in flatfoot reconstruction in children.

B

Bauman procedure, for calf contracture, 303
Bone disorders, navicular, flatfoot and, subtalar arthroereisis for, 326
Bunion(s), dorsal, 251
    treatment of, 260

C

Calcaneal stop procedure, for flatfoot, 320–321
Calf contracture, **301–306**
    pathomechanics of, 301–302
    treatment of
        nonoperative, 302
        surgical, 301–305
            Bauman procedure in, 303
            complications of, 305

Foot Ankle Clin N Am 15 (2010) 383–389
doi:10.1016/S1083-7515(10)00042-2
1083-7515/10/$ – see front matter © 2010 Elsevier Inc. All rights reserved.

foot.theclinics.com

Calf (*continued*)

      results of, 305

      Strayer procedure in, 303–304

      Vulpius procedure in, 304

Children

  clubfoot in

      residual, **245–264**. See also *Clubfoot, residual, in children.*

      treatment of, **235–243**. See also *Clubfoot, in infants and children, treatment of.*

    flatfoot in, management of, **309–322**. See also *Flatfoot, in children, management of.*

    foot and ankle disorders in, management of, gait analysis in, **364–382**. See also *Gait analysis, in foot and ankle disorders management, in children.*

Clubfoot

  in infants and children

    causes of, 235–236

    treatment of, **235–243**

      functional method in, 239

      historical background of, 236–237

      Ponseti technique in, 236–239

      surgical, 239–241

  overcorrection of, flatfoot secondary to, subtalar arthroereisis for, 326

  residual, in children, **245–264**

    causes of, 247–251

    deformities associated with, 247–251

      combined correction of, 260–261

      dorsal bunion, 251

      dynamic supination, 249

      forefoot adduction, 249

      intoeing gait, 250

      overcorrection, 250

      residual cavus, 249

      residual equinus, 247–249

      residual heel varus, 249

      rotary subluxation of navicular, 250–251

      treatment of, 253–260. See also specific deformities, e.g., *Residual equinus.*

    evaluation of, 251–253

    pathoanatomy of, 246–247

    treatment of, 253–260

      described, 245–246

      triple arthrodesis in, 261

  treated, adult sequelae of, **287–296**

    arthritis, 294

    clinical presentation of, 292–293

    concurrent degenerative conditions, 294–295

    described, 287–290

    evaluation and diagnosis of, 290–292

    overcorrection, 293

    undercorrection, 293

Computed tomography (CT)

  in residual clubfoot evaluation in children, 251–252

  in tarsal coalition, 355–356

Congenital talipes equinovarus (CTEV), relapsed or neglected, 265–267

Contracture(s), calf, **301–306.** See also *Calf contracture.*
CT. See *Computed tomography (CT).*
CTEV. See *Congenital talipes equinovarus (CTEV).*

D

Dorsal bunion, 251
   treatment of, 260
Dynamic supination, 249
   treatment of, 258

E

Endorthesis, in flatfoot reconstruction in children, 329
Evans procedure, for flatfoot, 316–319

F

Flatfoot
   clubfoot overcorrection and, subtalar arthroereisis for, 326
   described, 309–310
   flexible, subtalar arthroereisis for, 325–326
   in children
      background of, 310
      examination in, 310–311
      management of, **309–322**
         nonsurgical, 313–314
         surgical, 314–321
            calcaneal stop procedure in, 320–321
            described, 323–324
            Evans procedure in, 316–319
            lateral column lengthening in, 316–319
            medial calcaneal translational osteotomy in, 315–316
            medial cuneiform osteotomy in, 319–320
            subtalar arthroereisis in, **323–335.** See also *Subtalar arthroereisis, in flatfoot reconstruction in children.*
      patient history in, 310–311
      radiology of, 311–313
   navicular bone disorders with, subtalar arthroereisis for, 326
   spastic paralytic, subtalar arthroereisis for, 326
   tarsal coalition–related, subtalar arthroereisis for, 326
Foot and ankle deformities
   classification of, 268–269
   common conditions, 265–268
   compensatory mechanisms, 268
   severe, Ilizarov external fixation in correction of, **265–285.** See also *Ilizarov external fixation, in correction of severe pediatric foot and ankle deformities.*
Foot and ankle disorders, in children, management of, gait analysis in, **364–382.** See also *Gait analysis, in foot and ankle disorders management, in children.*
Foot motion, dynamic assessment of, 365–368
Forefoot adduction, 249
   treatment of, 258–259

G

Gait, intoeing, 250
    treatment of, 259
Gait analysis
    in foot and ankle disorders management, in children, **364–382**
        dynamic assessment in, 365–368
        kinematic foot models in
            development of, 368–379
            types of, 369–379
        OFM, 369–379. See also *Oxford Foot Model (OFM), in foot and ankle disorders management, in children.*
    in residual clubfoot evaluation in children, 252

I

Idiopathic toe walking, **297–300**
    differential diagnosis of, 297–298
    management of, 298
        literature review of, 298–300
    pathophysiology of, 297–298
    presentation of, 297
Ilizarov external fixation, in correction of severe pediatric foot and ankle deformities, **265–285**
    complications of, 277–279
    literature review related to, 279–282
    method of, 269
    operative technique, 273–276
        Ilizarov frame in, 273–275
        Taylor spatial frame in, 275–276
    postoperative care, 276–277
    preoperative assessment in, 272–273
    principles of, 269–271
    strategies in, 269–271
Ilizarov frame, in Ilizarov external fixation in correction of severe pediatric foot and ankle deformities, 273–275
Infant(s), clubfoot in, treatment of, **235–243**. See also *Clubfoot, in infants and children, treatment of.*
Intoeing gait, 250
    treatment of, 259

J

Joint injections, in residual clubfoot evaluation in children, 253

K

Kinematic foot models, development of, in foot and ankle disorders management, in children, 368–379

L

Lateral column lengthening, for flatfoot, 316–319
Lesser toes, treatment of, 260

M

Magnetic resonance imaging (MRI), in tarsal coalition, 356–357
Medial calcaneal translational osteotomy, for flatfoot, 315–316
Medial cuneiform osteotomy, for flatfoot, 319–320
Medial midfoot pain, differential diagnosis of, 340
Midfoot pain, medial, differential diagnosis of, 340
MRI. See Magnetic resonance imaging (MRI).

N

Navicular(s)
    accessory, **337–347**. See also Accessory naviculars (ANs).
    rotary subluxation of, 250–251
        treatment of, 259–260
Navicular bone disorders, flatfoot and, subtalar arthroereisis for, 326
Nuclear imaging, in tarsal coalition, 357

O

Osteotomy
    medial calcaneal translational, for flatfoot, 315–316
    medial cuneiform, for flatfoot, 319–320
Overcorrection
    as adult sequela of treated clubfoot, 293
    clubfoot and, 250
        treatment of, 259
Oxford Foot Model (OFM), in foot and ankle disorders management, in children, 369–379
    clinical use of, 374–379
    described, 369–369, 373–374

P

Pedobarography, in residual clubfoot evaluation in children, 252–253
Pes planus, in children, management of, **309–322**. See also Flatfoot, in children, management of.

R

Radiography
    in residual clubfoot evaluation in children, 251
    in tarsal coalition, 353–355
Radiology, in flatfoot evaluation, 311–313
Residual cavus, 249
    treatment of, 2567–258

Residual equinus
    in children, 247–249
    treatment of, 253, 255
Residual heel varus, 249
    treatment of, 255–256
Rotary subluxation of navicular, 250–251
    treatment of, 259–260

S

Sinus tarsi implant, subtalar arthroereisis with, in flatfoot reconstruction in children,
    324–325
Spastic paralytic flatfoot, subtalar arthroereisis for, 326
Strayer procedure, for calf contracture, 303–304
Subtalar arthroereisis, in flatfoot reconstruction in children, **323–335**
    complications of, 326–327
    discussion of, 333
    indications for, 325–326
    surgical technique, 327–329
        endorthesis, 329
        results of, 329–333
    with sinus tarsi implant, 324–325

T

Tarsal coalition, **349–364**
    causes of, 350–351
    complications of, 360
    flatfoot and, subtalar arthroereisis for, 326
    historical review of, 349–350
    imaging of, 353–357
        conventional radiography in, 353–355
        CT in, 355–356
        MRI in, 356–357
        nuclear imaging in, 357
    incidence of, 350
    management of, 357–360
        described, 357–358
        nonoperative, 358
        outcome of, 360
        postoperative, 359–360
        salvage surgery in, 359
        surgical, 358–359
    pathophysiology of, 351–352
    presentation of, 352–353
    prognosis, 360
Taylor spatial frame, in Ilizarov external fixation in correction of severe pediatric foot
    and ankle deformities, 275–276
Toe(s), lesser, treatment of, 260
Toe walking, idiopathic, **297–300.** See also *Idiopathic toe walking.*
Triceps surae, contracture of, **301–306.** See also *Calf contracture.*
Triple arthrodesis, for clubfoot, 261

U

Undercorrection, as adult sequela of treated clubfoot, 293

V

Vulpius procedure, for calf contracture, 304

Moving?

Make sure your subscription moves with you!

To notify us of your new address, find your **Clinics Account Number** (located on your mailing label above your name), and contact customer service at:

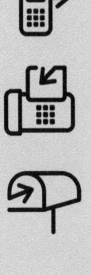

Email: journalscustomerservice-usa@elsevier.com

800-654-2452 (subscribers in the U.S. & Canada)
314-447-8871 (subscribers outside of the U.S. & Canada)

Fax number: 314-447-8029

Elsevier Health Sciences Division
Subscription Customer Service
3251 Riverport Lane
Maryland Heights, MO 63043

Printed and bound by CPI Group (UK) Ltd, Croydon, CR0 4YY

14/10/2024

01773708-0001